The Ageless Exercise Plan
A Complete Guide to Fitness After Fifty

Dr. Charles Godfrey
Michael Feldman

McGraw-Hill Book Company
New York   St. Louis   San Francisco   Bogotá   Guatemala
Hamburg   Lisbon   Madrid   Mexico   Panama
Paris   San Juan   São Paulo   Tokyo

Reprinted by arrangement with Key Porter Books
First McGraw-Hill Paperback edition, 1985.

1 2 3 4 5 6 7 8 9   8 7 6 5

This book is not meant to replace the services of a physician. Any application of the recommendations set forth in the following pages is at the reader's discretion and sole risk.

Library of Congress Cataloging in Publication Data

Godfrey, Charles M.
    The ageless exercise plan.

Reprint. Originally published: Key Porter Books, 1982.
1. Exercise for the aged.   2. Exercise therapy.
3. Physical fitness.   4. Aged — Health and hygiene.
I. Feldman, Michael.   II. Title.

RA781.6.G64 1984   613.7'1   84-20186
ISBN 0-07-023629-1 (pbk.)

Design: Fortunato Aglialoro (Studio 2 Graphics)
Photography: Jeremy Jones
Typesetting: Compeer Typographic Services Limited
Printing and Binding: Gagné Printing Ltd.
Chairs courtesy of Eaton's
Printed and bound in Canada

Contents

Introduction 4
1 The Exercise Bonus 5
2 How Fit Are You? 9
3 Get Ready, Get Set, Go 15
4 Basic Ageless Exercises 22
5 Alternate Ageless Exercises 35
6 Advanced Ageless Exercises 47
7 The Problem Exerciser 63
8 Lifestyle Activities 83
Progress Charts 91
About the Authors 95

Introduction

The Ageless Exercise Plan is an exercise guide for those of the over-fifty population who are anxious to regain healthy levels of physical fitness and activity. Its main emphasis is the development of joint flexibility and muscle power sufficient for the specific demands which you make on your body. Its premise is that muscle power without joint flexibility can be self-defeating. Its message is *All that is required is twenty minutes of energetic exercise, three times a week, plus a few minutes of stretching exercises each day.* Its warning is *Don't hurt yourself, exercise in a safe, sane way for the rest of your long, long life.*

1
THE EXERCISE BONUS

So you want to get fit! You've finally decided that you've put it off for too many days, and you realize that unless something is done about it right now, it's going to be twenty times harder farther down the road. Great!

Physical fitness can increase your enjoyment of life, step up your appetite, make you look better and keep you out of the sick bed. Most people know that, but older people (let's get this clear: older in age, not necessarily in spirit) somehow never get around to a regular exercise program.

They may exercise on the weekend or sporadically one or two times a week. Or they may wait until they go away to the cottage and try to get back into shape there. Or they may spend a lot of money enrolling in a health club, only to drop out. Sound familiar? The startling fact is that most people do not have a regular exercise plan which they intend to continue for the rest of their lives.

That's sad, because exercising is easy to do, can become an enjoyable habit and can make you look and feel better than you ever did before. And you don't have to spend a lot of time, or exhaust or hurt yourself. You can forget all those visions you have of groaning bodies or pavement-pounding joggers.

The first thing to remember is that your age is no barrier to fitness. Scientific studies have shown that even inactive men and women in their eighties and nineties can greatly improve their mental and physical health with exercise! Regular physical activity can compensate for the normal functional changes that occur with increasing age. And in many cases, the commonly accepted loss of strength in older people may not be due to the aging process, but rather to lack of activity.

Inactivity can reduce physical fitness abilities. However, four months of an exercise program can increase your exercise capacity in the same way it can increase that of younger men and women. In addition, exercise can decrease your blood pressure, improve your heart rate and increase your flexibility. Unlike many of the machines in our society, the human body is not designed to deteriorate on schedule. So forget those TV commercials that stress your age but not your ability!

Perhaps your problem has been getting around to exercising. And perhaps you have some reason to fret because you've tried before and it didn't work. Let's look at why it didn't work. Most likely you set a goal that was simply too high. While physical activity can make you younger, fresher and more vibrant, it can't turn you into a Wayne Gretzky. So, set a realistic goal. As a matter of fact, a series of goals. The first one you reach in four months, the next one in twelve months, the next one beyond that figure. But the main thing is to set a goal and have a plan to reach it. We'll show you how to organize such a plan in Chapter 3.

Or maybe you've compared yourself with somebody else and have given up. Jennie, who lives next door, jogs eight miles a day and drives you mad with her constant burble about breaking the barrier or hitting the wall. This can be upsetting when you can barely manage to get down to the corner and back to pick up a carton of milk. Well, don't compare yourself with her. Pick your own program, walk your own mile and gradually increase your activity, regardless of the rest of the world.

Then, there is always the problem of time. Where are you

going to find the hours to do all this? Physical fitness demands a great deal of time — you know that because you've seen the hours all those other people put into it. Now let's be reasonable. Three 20-minute periods of energetic exercise per week plus some specific stretching exercises each day can keep anybody fit. Add a good diet and you can skip through life. That's a pretty small investment when you consider how much time you really do have.

Of course, it's necessary to actually do the exercises. Robert Benchley used to say that every time he felt like doing an exercise, he lay down until the thought left. That was a great line, but the truth is that he kept himself very busy with a general activity program. The secret is to schedule your time. Get into the habit of exercising and you'll reach your fitness goal.

What is the benefit of all this? Will you really have more energy, look better, feel younger, have more self-confidence, feel less tense? No doubt about it! And it's all there as a reward for picking a reasonable program, staying with it and enjoying it.

"But," you say, "I look sort of silly doing those exercises when I'm in the shape I'm in. All the pictures I see in the how-to books show a slim, beautiful person, like Jane Fonda, doing sit-ups. I couldn't manage that and besides, I sag here and there . . ." Come off it. Nobody cares what you look like when you exercise except you. Besides, most people exercise in private. Even if you do join a group, there most likely will be some very friendly people who will be supportive, uncritical and a great help. Don't pull a bag over your head as you go into the gym; just keep your eye on the fact that four months down the road you'll be a new person.

Don't forget the others in your family. Include them in your exercise plan. Maybe they will want to join you. Certainly, if you are going to do a general physical activity program, you'd better go public with your plans and explain to family and friends what's going on. Your broadcast can lead to all kinds of support springing up from various places, including your neighbors, the "Y" just around the corner, a "Second Mile Club" or a volunteer group.

Why has it taken you this long to get to this stage? When are you going to bite the bullet and get fit? Why, if all of the above is true, has it taken you this long to say "That's for me"? Maybe you've noticed it's harder work to do the same thing today than when you did it a year ago. You're breathing more heavily. Maybe your heart is pumping a little harder and a little faster than it did before. Or you're a little clumsy while walking on the street. Maybe there isn't the old zip that you used to have. You can leave all those complaints behind and go on to a new level of living with the Ageless Exercise Plan.

2
HOW FIT ARE YOU?

Just as starting a long trip demands some planning, you should make up a check list of how you stack up in the fitness area before you start your exercise program.

Checking with Your Doctor

Most people know whether they should start a physical fitness program. However, because this is a sane program, if you have heart trouble, or pains in your head or chest, or feel faint, or have spells of severe dizziness, check with your physician before you start into the muscle business. Similarly, if you are under treatment for, say, high blood pressure or have bone or joint problems such as arthritis, which could be aggravated by exercise, check with your friendly family doc as to how he or she feels about your joining the Ageless Exercise Plan.

Does your doctor think you should be doing unrestricted physical activity? Should you be under some supervision to meet the specific needs that you have? Or should you just forget the whole idea?

If none of these problems affect you, then by all means let's get started on a graduated exercise plan. The only thing stopping you will be a temporary minor illness, such as a cold or some gastro-intestinal upset. If this happens, ease off on the exercises for a few days until it passes.

Checking Your Flexibility and Energy Fitness

There are three types of fitness. The most common type is energy fitness: having enough get up and go in your body to carry out everyday activities. In addition, there should be a little to spare to make sure that when you sprint for the bus, you won't be running for an ambulance. *Energy fit* is the same thing as *aerobic fit*. It is the result of exercises that increase the strength of your muscles, reduce your heart rate and increase your lung capacity. More oxygen gets to your muscles, and they use it more efficiently, with less waste products.

The second type of fitness is flexibility fitness. *Flexibility fit* means that the joints go through a good range of movement, enabling you to use the dynamo-like muscles that you are developing to their best advantage. Lack of flexibility can mean that a good deal of the energy fitness you have created is not delivered. You get muscle-bound.

And the third type of fitness is the one that goes with the mind. This is the emotional position you take when faced with the opportunity to do physical activities. It helps to decide that activity and exercise are fun — instead of dodging activity, you feel so good you go out searching for it. You actually enjoy "working out." It's great for your enjoyment of life — all phases of life — and it makes you think more clearly. The exercises in this book involve all three types of fitness.

Now before you get out there and recall how it was when you were twenty-nine, here are one or two things you should know. Your muscles may have lost some of their strength, power and endurance due to lack of use. Naturally this affects their function, so they may not respond as you expect.

Additionally, the articular cartilage (the shiny stuff seen in the leg of a chicken), which allows that nice, smooth bending of the knee when you squat, may be frayed and pitted. There may be a little grinding when you bend your knees.

And on trying to squat, you may notice that the flexibility of your knees and ankles isn't what it used to be. In addition to feeling stiff, you realize that you can't do all of those movements that the young person does on the TV show. This decrease in mobility may also be combined with some instability — you tend to fall off to one side. That knee, which has walked a million miles, occasionally seems to buckle.

Don't be alarmed or discouraged. It's natural, and there is something that can be done to remedy all of these problems. Of course, if you begin to exercise vigorously without building up to it, your joints will not be protected against overload and there will be trouble. Remember to be safe and sane.

Let's begin by measuring your flexibility. As you do the flexibility exercises, keep a record of your progress (see page 19). The main target areas to keep loose are the knees, ankles, shoulders, hips, neck and back.

First, the knees.

- *Begin gently to test their flexibility by squatting slowly between two chairs, using your arms to control the descent.*

- *To increase the flexibility of your knees, do this exercise five times and then stop.*

You'll find out tonight or tomorrow morning that there is a slight feeling of stiffness around the knees. But practice this exercise for a week or ten days and — eureka! — you will actually be able to squat down fully, where before it was impossible.

However, if there has been previous injury in this region, you may find that the movements are not smooth, rather they tend to clunk along. If your knee grinds and bucks as you bend it, try to move the joint without the full weight of your body bearing down on the area. Or even better, see if you can separate the two joint surfaces. This can be done, for example in the knee, by sitting on the edge of a table and letting the leg hang freely. Fasten a weight cuff of approximately four pounds to your ankle.

You'll notice that the leg tends to pull out of the knee socket. Swing the leg back and forth slowly and see if you can get a greater range of movement. You can do the same activity with the shoulders or hips by fastening the weight cuff to your arm or lower thigh. This increased range of movement can usually get around the particular problem of cracking or fraying of the articular cartilage and get you back on the exercise track.

To measure the flexibility of your neck:

- *Lie on your back on the floor and turn your head to the right.*

- *Measure how many degrees of movement your head goes through from an imaginary upright line which is zero degrees. If you can turn your head all the way over to the right, that's ninety degrees. Repeat on the left side.*

Next, let's look at your shoulders.

- *While still on your back with elbows tucked into your side and arms upright, let the right arm sink outwards towards the floor.*

- *Once again calculate the number of degrees between the upright starting position (zero degrees) and the end point. Then do the same with the left arm. Young people should be able to touch their arm to the floor. That's ninety degrees. In older people the movement may be a good deal less.*

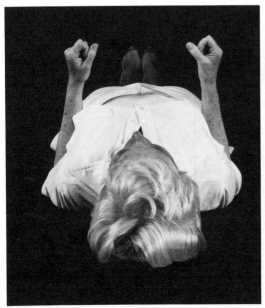
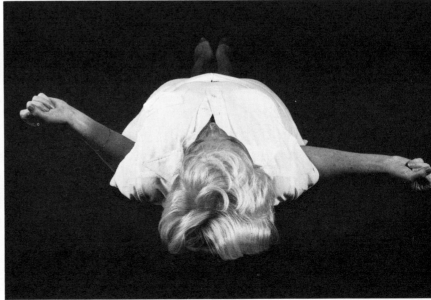

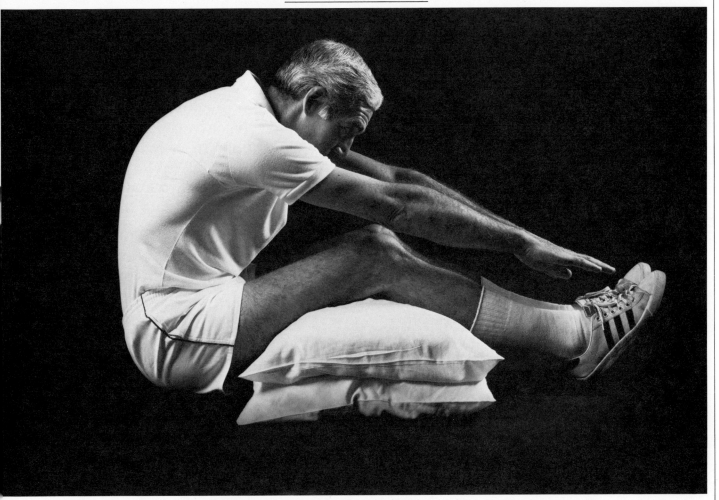

⇪ Now measure lumbar spine flexibility.

- *While still on your back put a pillow beneath your knees so that they are bent at an angle of about thirty degrees.*

- *Now bend your trunk forward so that your hands are going towards your toes.*

- *Measure the distance between your fingertips and your toes. The reason the knees have been bent is to compensate for those people who have short hamstrings and never could touch their toes. When you measure in this way, you get a true index of the flexibility of the back.*

And finally, test your hip joints.

- *While on your back, with the left leg straight out, measure how close your knee comes to your chest when you bend your right leg up as far as you can.*

- *Then test your left hip joint in the same way.*

In addition to flexibility fitness, you're aiming for energy fitness, and this is measured by pulse rate. To check your resting pulse rate, take it first thing in the morning when you wake up. The lower it is, the better for you. Pulse rates can be taken at the wrist by placing the middle three fingers of the right hand along the edge of the wrist of the left arm just below the base of the thumb. You can also take your pulse by pressing alongside the Adam's apple in your throat, but don't be overly vigorous in pressing on this point, because it can cause some dizziness.

Checking Your Weight

Don't forget to weigh yourself regularly every week. This helps you to remember that exercise and weight go together. Measure your body fat by picking up the skin on your abdomen between the thumb and index finger and sensing how much blubber is present. More than one inch is too much.

You now know how flexible you are. You know your energy fitness level from your heart rate and you have a baseline measure of weight. Let's see how you can change those measurements with the Ageless Exercise Plan.

3
GET READY, GET SET, GO

The Ageless Exercise Plan's basic principle is if you don't use it, you'll lose it. No matter how you interpret "it," most people like to hang on to it.

Dressing for the Occasion

Now that you've made the decision to exercise, you'd better dress for the occasion.

We suggest you wear loose, light, comfortable clothing so that you can keep mobile. Use firm shoes with a soft non-skid sole. Running shoes are fine. If the breasts are heavy and pendulous, wear a strong brassiere. Those are the sensible suggestions. But, if you want to doll-up and wear one of those jazzy jogging suits or a leotard, go right ahead. Just make sure it's washable, because before long you're going to perspire. On the other hand, a cotton shirt and a pair of slacks or shorts will give you all the covering you need and help you to stay within your budget.

Simple Equipment

You don't need any special equipment to start on our exercise adventure. A small rubber ball is used in a few exercises. It also helps to have a strong chair, preferably wood, with non-skid feet and no arms. A large clock with a second sweep hand is handy to time your pulse and the activity period. A simple weight cuff, which you can put on your ankle or arm, is useful for the flexibility test in Chapter 2 and for advanced exercises, but not absolutely necessary.

Beware of the advertisements that seduce you with magic mechanical shortcuts to fitness. Electrical gadgets, mini-gyms — forget them! A safe, sane exercise formula uses your two arms, two legs and what's between the ears. There's more bunk written about home exercise equipment than there is on hair restorers or detergents.

Time to Have Fun

The best time to exercise is the time most convenient to you. It's important, however, to schedule your exercise period; do it at the same time each day and establish a regular routine. Avoid exercise immediately after meals. Go through the entire basic exercise plan at least three times per week when starting and then, when you are comfortable with your program (after four to six weeks), you can make it part of your daily routine.

If, for some reason, you can't exercise every day, don't worry. According to the experts, exercising until you are out of breath for twenty minutes, three times a week, will help you achieve a good level of energy fitness. And if your joints go through a full range of movement once per day, that's enough for flexibility fitness.

Begin your program gradually. Start with ten minutes of exercise and then increase to a comfortable twenty to thirty minutes. Usually you should do three complete repetitions of each exercise. Exceptions to this rule are noted in the guide.

Remember, this is a safe, sane plan. Don't push yourself too heavily. If yesterday's exercise left you a little stiff, that's great. But you should have been back to your normal self in a few hours. If you felt pooped all day, then you were too hearty. Be sane and reduce the effort a bit today. Most people who give up this healthy activity do so because they overdo it and injure themselves. The fitness movement has hit our society in the same way hula-hoops and yo-yos did. There are a lot of people out there making a buck out of persuading you to do more. Ignore them. Save your money and your health by doing what is sufficient to maintain your fitness.

Warm Up, Cool Down

As all good drivers know, a car's engine should be warmed up before the car is driven. You should do the same. Your exercise warm-up is not only a matter of increasing circulation to your muscles, but is also a gradual stretching of muscles so that you don't tear any tissues at the beginning of your program. It's a safety factor.

Begin each session by breathing deeply. More people achieve a feeling of well-being from good breathing habits than any other physical activity. If you sit around all day, you most likely use slightly more than one-tenth of a cubic foot of air a minute. But to feel and think brightly you should be gulping at least one cubic foot for a short time.

Similarly, at the end of the exercise period, cool down. When a thoroughbred completes the Kentucky Derby, a groom walks the horse for a good twenty minutes. The same applies when dealing with a thoroughbred like yourself. Observe the same cooling-down process to prevent muscle soreness and to promote relaxation and the feeling of well-being that comes from exercising.

Doing the Ageless Exercises

There are several ways of doing an exercise. We'll use your biceps as a model. The description uses words that are pretty fancy but go along with the directions and it will be quite clear.

- *Bend your right arm in towards your face to make a ninety-degree angle.*
- *Put your left hand on the inside of your right wrist.*

- *Pull the right hand towards the nose, resisting slightly with the left hand.*

This is called an isotonic exercise; the pressure inside your right bicep remains about the same, but the length of the muscle shortens.

- *Now take up the same position with the left hand pressing against the right wrist, but this time increase the resistance of the left hand to the right elbow which is flexing.*
- *Stop the elbow from flexing and put out as much of a push as you can to overcome the flexing of your right arm.*

This is called an isometric exercise. That is, the length of the muscle remains the same (the arm doesn't move), but the pressure changes.

So you have isometric and isotonic. Notice the word *iso* is there all the time. It means maintaining the same level. *Tonic* means pressure inside the muscle, and *metric* means length.

In addition to these two methods of muscle building, there is a further division.

- *Again, place your left hand on your right wrist.*
- *Pull the right hand towards your nose.*

When you move closer to the nose, that is called a concentric exercise. The biceps muscle is shortening or contracting.

- *Now start again with the right elbow bent at right angles and the left hand on the right wrist.*
- *With the left hand push the elbow out straight, resisting at the same time by contracting the biceps.*

Note that the biceps are elongating, not getting shorter. This is called an eccentric exercise. The muscle contracts, but gets longer.

All this description isn't intended to foster the use of Latin in your daily life. There are advantages in using each type of exercise. For example, isometric exercises have been used throughout history to build muscles of great power. Theseus, a

Greek warrior, was said to have lifted a calf each morning before breakfast. As the calf grew larger, Theseus became more powerful. Finally, when Theseus was full grown, he was lifting a bull.

That may sound like a lot of bull to you, but muscles can be built to an enormous size and strength. The principle used by Theseus was a gradual increase of effort on a daily basis. As most farmers know, a calf usually puts on one pound of weight per day. So Theseus was increasing his work output by this amount every day and eventually became a big-time weight-lifter. You don't want to go that far. But with a small increase in resistance every day, you too can be like a Greek god — or at least able to lift your body out of bed, carry the groceries and enjoy physical activities.

When doing the exercises, you will sometimes see the term *bounce it*. This tells you that the motion in the exercise should be pushed a little more, then relaxed, then pushed again, to stretch the tissues.

Most exercises are done to a time count of "one thousand and one." If the instruction is "Hold for a count of two," that means "one thousand and one, one thousand and two."

Remember. Don't be afraid to take a break between each exercise. Don't push yourself if you feel tired. Use the professional slogan "Train, don't strain."

Keeping a Progress Chart

The chart in the back of this book will help you keep track of your progress in the next four months. It's divided into three sections: Flexibility Exercises (Exercises 2, 3, 4, 5, 6, 8, 9, 10, 13, 15, 17, 18, 20, 22, 25, 26, 30), Energy Exercises (Exercises 7, 14, 16, 19, 21, 23, 24, 27, 28, 29 and the activities in Chapter 8) and Special Exercises for the Problem Exerciser (Exercises 31, 32, 33, 34, 35, 36, 37, 38, 39, 40, 41, 42).

Begin by following the Basic Ageless Exercises in Chapter 4. See Chapter 5 for Alternate Ageless Exercises. Flexibility exercises for your neck, arms, shoulders, back, hands, waist, legs and feet should be done each day. Enter the numbers of the ones you do and measure your flexibility at the beginning and end of the week (page 11). The special exercises should also be done daily.

You should "train" three times a week by doing the Basic or Alternate energy exercises. As you increase your level of energy fitness, your resting heart rate will decrease. Another way to measure your progress is to clock how long it takes to walk 100 feet. As you become more fit, the elapsed time will decrease.

The resting heart rate gives you a good idea of your progress. In order to make that progress, you must exercise at a training rate. Usually you should be training at 120 beats per minute. If you exercise at too low a rate, then the energy fitness level will not be raised. If, on the other hand, the heart rate is too high, say 140, then you are not practicing a safe, sane program. Any warm-up exercise will raise the heart rate, so when you're into the exercise, check the rate for ten seconds and compare it with the desired heart rate level.

Once you're at the desired level, then your session should continue for at least fifteen minutes to get the training effect. However, don't forget, you are in training. To begin with, stay at that level for only two to three minutes and then gradually increase the length of time at that level of activity.

In addition to the Basic or Alternate energy exercises, you can use the flexibility exercises for energy purposes, as long as your heart rate is at the desired level. After four months, you'll be ready to go on to the more energetic Advanced Ageless Exercises combined with other activities (see Chapter 8).

Keep the plan in an easy-to-read place alongside your exercise area. Your progress chart can be cut out and mounted on the wall or spread out so that you can enter your activities from day to day.

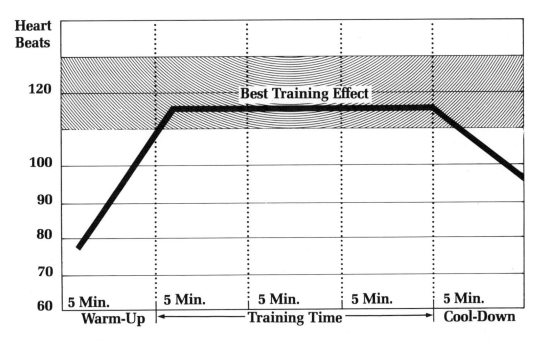

HEART RATE

At the end of your exercise session, check how long it takes for your heart rate to return to normal. As your level of fitness increases, the time decreases.

Exercising Alone or with Friends

You may find that your progress chart is full for the first few weeks and then becomes spotty. Don't give up! If you are alone, we suggest you do the exercises to music. Or why not exercise with a friend or form your own fitness group? The only thing to watch is that you don't lose some of the safety aspects of the exercises by competing with your neighbor. Keep any competition at the fun level.

Fitness classes are recommended. They give plenty of support to each of the participants, and there is usually an instructor who can ensure that you are following your plan in a safe, sane manner. This type of supervision can be helpful. If it isn't available to you, then send your questions to us and we will try to answer them for you.

4
BASIC AGELESS EXERCISES

Feeling relaxed and having a sufficient supply of oxygen are necessary in any fitness plan. By doing some simple breathing exercises prior to exercising you can increase the supply of oxygen which is necessary for energy. As you become more fit, you will find you can do more work with less oxygen. That's when you begin to experience the first real benefit from all that work!

1 Breathing Exercise

Each deep breath is a deposit in the bank of health and gives you a feeling of well-being. Do this exercise as part of any warm-up. Try it when the window is open. Inhale cool air and lay in a little capital for your next "all-out" effort.

- *With your arms in front of your body and with fingertips meeting, raise your hands slowly straight over your head.*
- *Inhale through the nose while raising.*
- *Then, while exhaling through the mouth, lower your arms to the starting position.*
- *Make sure that you take a deep breath in and then exhale it completely with a little cough at the end of the exhalation, just to make sure all the air is blown out.*
- *Do it five times to the rhythm of "The Blue Danube" or any other waltz.*

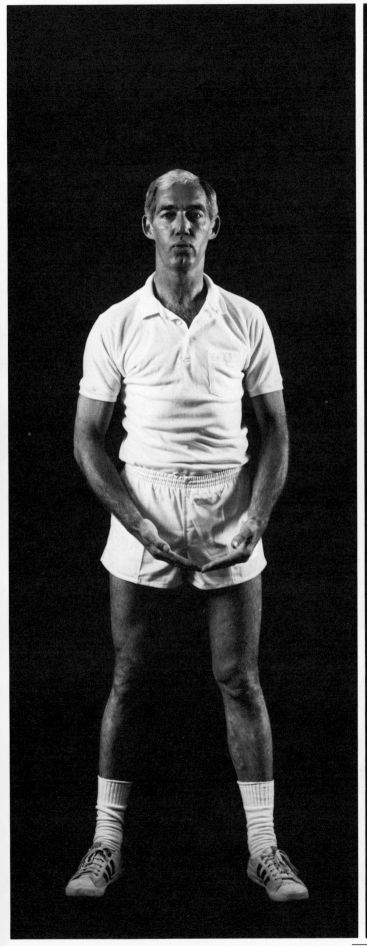
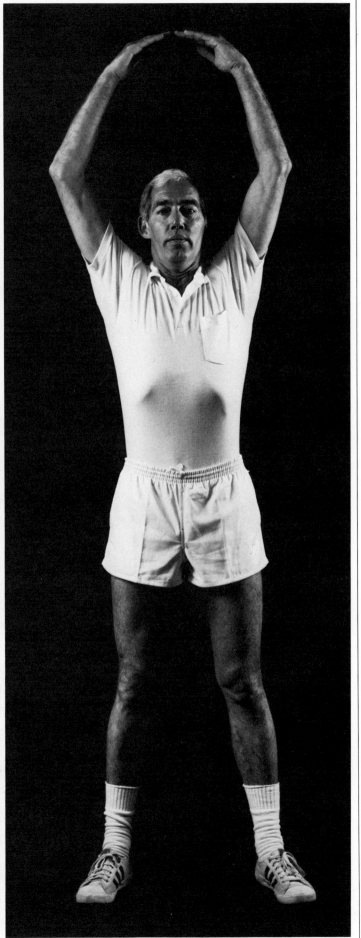

2 Neck Mobility Exercise

Earlier we talked about the necessity of maintaining a full range of movement in all your joints. This applies particularly to the neck. Many adults complain of neck stiffness, which can progress to neck pain and headaches. Regular exercises will preserve the flexibility of your neck and make it easier to look over your shoulder while backing up the car.

To maintain and improve both flexibility and range of motion in your neck do the following exercise:

- *Sit erect with your back and shoulders pressed into the back of a chair.*
- *Flex your head forward to your chest, then bring it back as slowly as possible as far as it will go.*
- *Return to the starting position.*
- *Now turn the head slowly to the left until your chin is over the shoulder and return to the starting position.*
- *Then turn to the right.*
- *Do this exercise three times.*

This exercise can be combined with breathing so that you exhale when you are lowering your head and inhale while raising it, inhale while turning the head away from the center line and exhale when returning it to the starting position.

Once again do these exercises slowly. If you find they cause any discomfort, particularly when looking at the ceiling, don't push yourself; simply go through the motion until it begins to feel uncomfortable and then ease off and return to the starting position. Sometimes you may notice some "clunking" as you go through the movements. Not to worry. That's just the result of getting it in the neck for forty years, and it will gradually quieten.

3 Shoulder Shrugs and Rotations

Many headaches and a general feeling of tightness and tension behind your ears are caused by failure of the muscles in the upper part of the back and lower portion of the neck. You can avoid these problems by doing shrugs and rotations.

- ◉ *While inhaling, slowly lift your left shoulder upwards to the ear.*
- ◉ *Then drop your shoulder and at the same time breathe out and relax.*
- ◉ *Once again with inhalation lift your right shoulder to the ear.*
- ◉ *Drop the shoulder, breathe out and relax. Just feel the muscles lengthen and relax.*
- ◉ *Now, while inhaling slowly lift both shoulders upward to the ears, like a turtle pulling its head into its shell.*

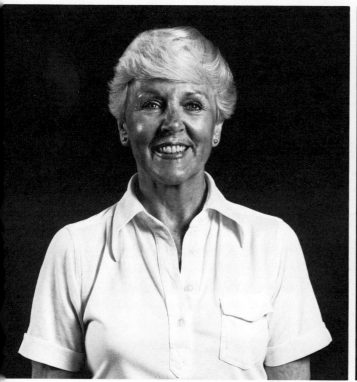 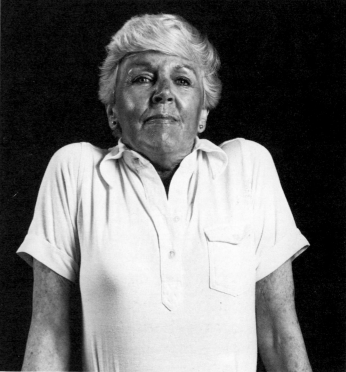

- ◉ *Drop your shoulders, breathe out and relax.*
- ◉ *To complete the shoulder exercises, rotate them in a forward motion in a circle. That is, bring both shoulders up and forward, down and back so that you end up making a full circle.*

- *Breathe in while lifting the shoulders and breathe out while lowering them. You can see how slowly this exercise has to be done otherwise you will be huffing and panting in quick order.*
- *Reverse the motion by rotating the shoulders backwards to start the circle.*
- *Now relax and take a deep breath.*
- *Do this series three times.*

4 Arm Rotations

A common problem you may experience is difficulty in putting on heavy coats or reaching to the back of the car to pick up a parcel. This is usually caused by loss of flexibility about the shoulder joint. The shoulder is a ball-and-socket joint and it is vital to maintain its free mobility. It can be done with this exercise.

- *Hold your arms out at your sides at shoulder height. You can do this while seated in a chair or standing.*
- *Now, start making small circles with the arms and slowly enlarge the circles until the arms are swinging in front of your body. This is done SLOWLY, in a controlled movement. Don't throw the arms about.*
- *When the circles are large enough that your hands are meeting in front of your body, then reverse and make smaller circles until you return to the starting position.*
- *Remember, this is an exercise and not a warm-up prior to taking off! Do it slowly three times.*

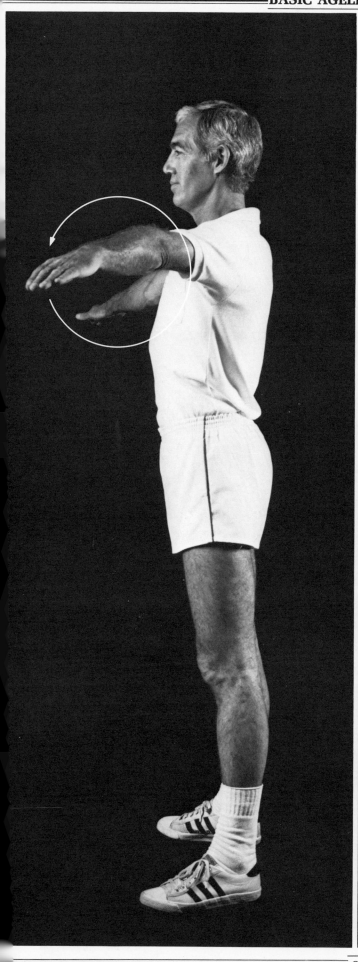
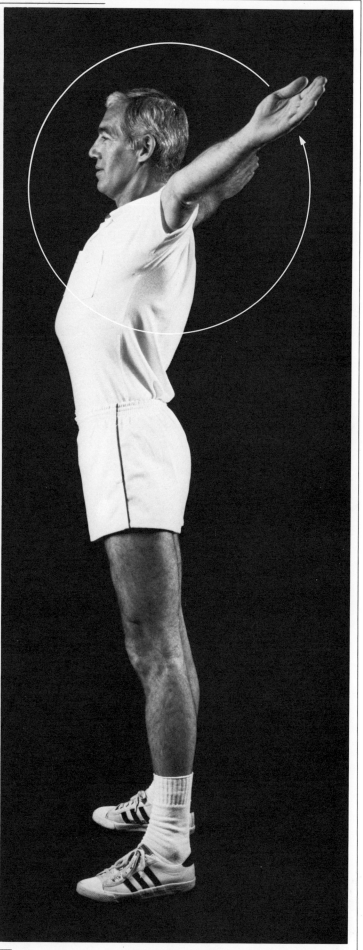

5 Feldman Punch and Squeeze

One of the big problems in our modern world is getting at our food. In addition to being expensive to buy, it's hard to open. We forget that it's also necessary to exercise our hands in order to keep them strong and flexible. The Feldman Punch is designed to make it easier to open those bottles, do the carpentry or just grab on for dear life.

- *Place your hands in front of your body, then reach out as far as you can.*
- *Make a tight fist, hold for five seconds, relax.*
- *Stretch out your fingers and wiggle them around. Make them dance.*
- *Do this exercise three times.*
- *To keep the fingers loose and strong, hold a rubber ball of about 2 1/2 inches diameter in your hand and squeeze it to the count of five.*
- *Relax. Repeat this concentric exercise until you can see the whites of your knuckles, then do it another five times.*

6 The Back Stretch

There is a special section in Chapter 7 for people with back pain. Although not everyone has a back problem, most of us need to do back exercises, particularly those which increase flexibility in the lower portion of the spine. Free, easy movement is one of the surest ways to keep out of the doctor's office.

- *Sit on your straight chair, and check your posture once per day by putting your feet flat on the floor and pressing the lower part of your spine into the back of the chair.*
- *At the same time imagine that you are being suspended by a few gray hairs of your head. This will pull the head up as high as it will go while the lower part of your back is still in contact with the chair's back.*
- *Now, slowly bend forward as close to the floor as possible and then straighten up to your previous posture.*

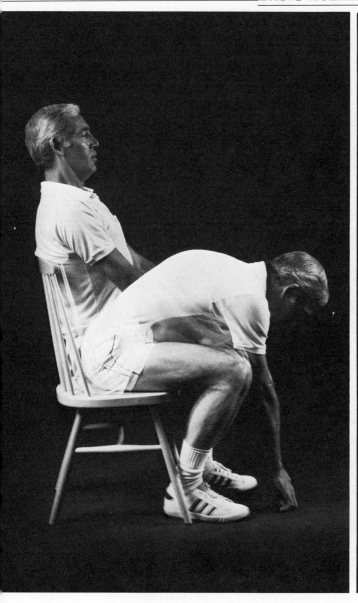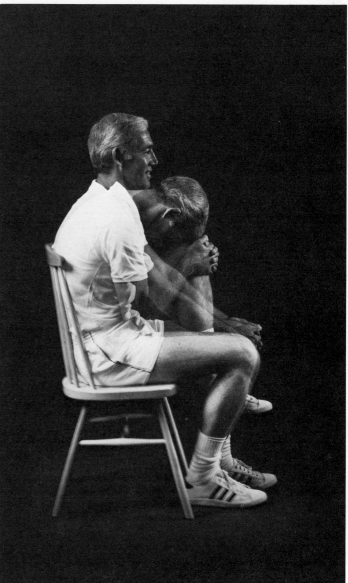

- Do this twice.

- Next, pull your left knee up to your chest with both hands and at the same time bend your head forward to meet your knee. You'll feel a little tug at your lower backside. That's good!

- Put your left knee back to the starting position and pull your right knee up in the same way.

- This gentle stretching exercise should be done twice in each session. Don't yank at your knee — just a slow, steady pull will be enough to stretch those tight hamstrings, the muscles at the back of your thighs.

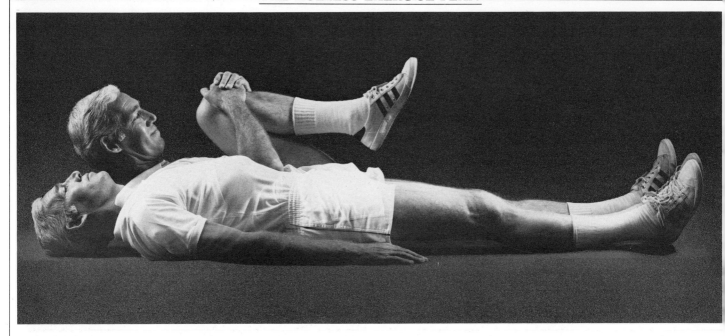

- *An alternate way to do this exercise is while you are lying flat on your back.*
- *Put your hands around one knee. With the other leg straight, pull the knee to your chest. At the same time, raise your head towards the knee.*
- *Hold for a count of two. Then do the same with the other leg.*
- *Do it five times.*

7 Waist and Stomach Strengthener

If you take care of your diet and exercise, there is no reason why your thyroid gland should slip down to your belt line causing a big bulge. A little exercise will keep your waist measurement at a reasonable level and at the same time protect your vanity and your back.

- *Sit on the front edge of a chair with your shoulders touching the backrest and your back held straight.*
- *Now move your legs in a pedaling fashion.*
- *Sing "A Bicycle Built For Two" and keep time for one minute.*
- *Start this exercise slowly and build up your endurance. Stop if you begin to feel tired or get a feeling of stress in your back.*

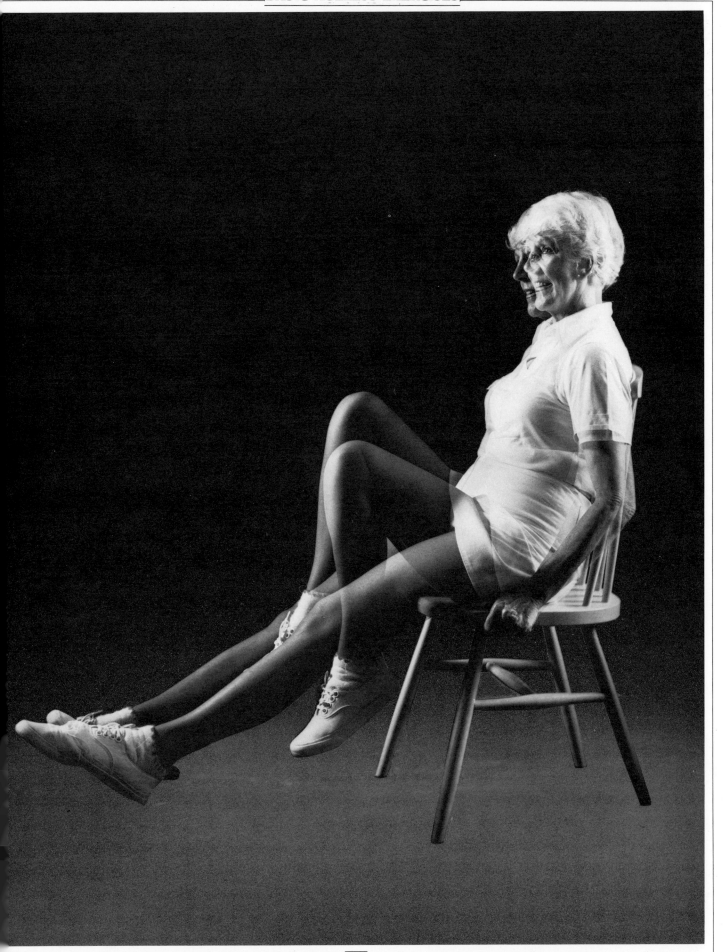

Your back's stability depends on a good set of abdominal muscles. Those are the ones you can feel if you try to blow out while you have closed your windpipe.

This exercise uses your hip flexors and your "kick" muscles, while at the same time your back is supporting the rest of your body. It is a concentric isotonic exercise for all these muscles.

8 Leg and Knee Lift

The previous exercise strengthens your back and the upper part of your legs. Here is one that works along the same lines. However, it stretches your muscles, making it easier to climb stairs or put on a brief spurt to catch a bus.

- ◉ *Sit straight back in your chair and point one leg out in front of you.*
- ◉ *Then slowly lift your entire leg up a few inches more and bend the toes towards the nose.*
- ◉ *Can you feel the pull in the back of your legs and on your bottom? This means you are stretching the muscles and that's good! Relax.*
- ◉ *Change legs and repeat twice.*

9 Knee Flexing

In Chapter 2, you read about testing the flexibility in your knees. That exercise is one of the Basic Ageless Exercises.

- ◉ *Stand between two chairs. While supporting some of your weight with your arms, bend the knees slowly.*
- ◉ *Squat five times, going down a little further each time.*

Never do this exercise without the chairs for support.

10 Foot Flexing

Moving up and down stairs or going to get the groceries involves your feet too. The problem with feet is that they are at the end of the body and so far away that you tend to forget them! There are 26 bones, 197 ligaments, 19 muscles and 33

joints in those structures which support you when standing. Imagine the forces that act through the foot while dancing, jumping, or simply trying to turn off the faucet while in the tub!

- ◉ *Still sitting in the chair put one leg straight out in front and point the toes down.*
- ◉ *Then pull them up towards your nose.*
- ◉ *Keep the leg straight.*
- ◉ *Rest and repeat with the opposite leg.*
- ◉ *Do it slowly so that you feel every motion of the ankle, without moving the leg.*
- ◉ *Point the toes as far to the east as you can and then to the north and then to the south and then to the west.*
- ◉ *You can do both feet together, and can go clockwise or counterclockwise.*
- ◉ *Relax when you feel a heavy pulling sensation.*
- ◉ *Make slow, circling movements five times in each direction.*

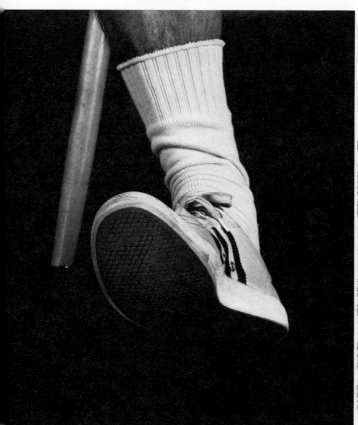
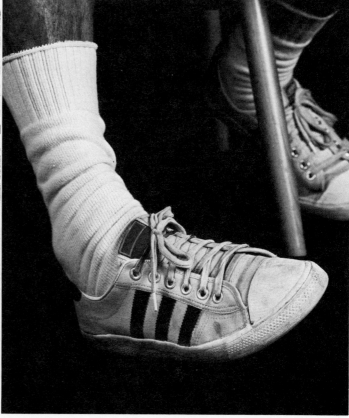

As one gets older, the ligaments in the feet tend to stretch slightly, which means that you are more prone to flat feet and other painful conditions. Doing foot exercises will help prevent you from ever saying "Oh, my aching feet!"

11 Cool It Exercise

This is a relaxing exercise to do as you are finishing up your session.

- *Sit cross-legged, or as close to it as you can, with your back straight.*
- *Stretch one arm up over your head to the ceiling and then let it drop into your lap.*
- *Repeat with the alternate arm, taking a deep breath as you raise the arm and breathing out completely as you lower it.*
- *Then look at your left leg and foot. Consciously will yourself to relax them, tighten a little, then relax again.*
- *You can do this deliberate tighten and relax sequence to any part of your body — especially to the furrowed brow!*

That is the basic part of the Ageless Exercise Plan. It can be done without hurting yourself, yet is good enough, combined with some other energy activity, to start you on the road to fitness.

Do you feel that something is missing? That it all sounds too easy? Is that really all that's required to reach the goal of fitness? The answer is "Yes, that's all you have to do!" Of course, if you enjoy it, do a lot more, but these general exercises are sufficient.

And don't let any of the hawkers of club memberships or the messiahs of marathon running tell you otherwise. Like vitamin pills, brown bread or sex, exercise has been blown out of proportion in Western society by the media. It's time you realized just how little effort or inconvenience there is in a safe, sane plan.

5
ALTERNATE
AGELESS EXERCISES

Because exercising can be dull, try different ways to get the same results. Here are some alternative flexibility and energy exercises. Choose the ones that you enjoy the most, but don't flit from one exercise to another. Keep the same alternates on at least a weekly basis.

Remember. Work slowly, stay within your limits and don't forget the deep breath and that big exhalation.

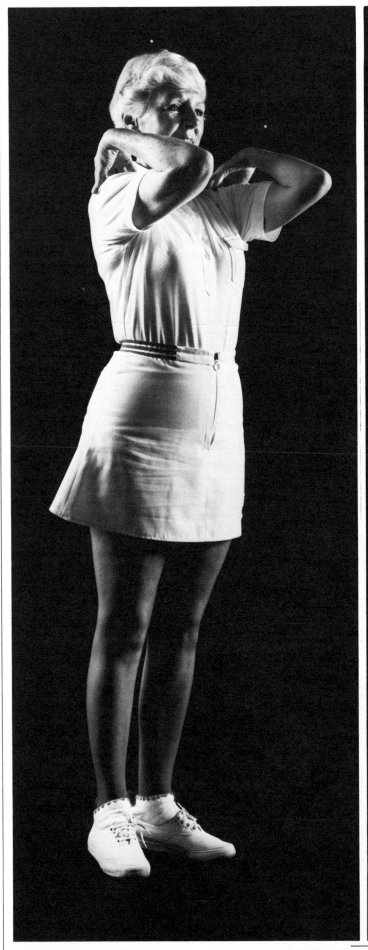 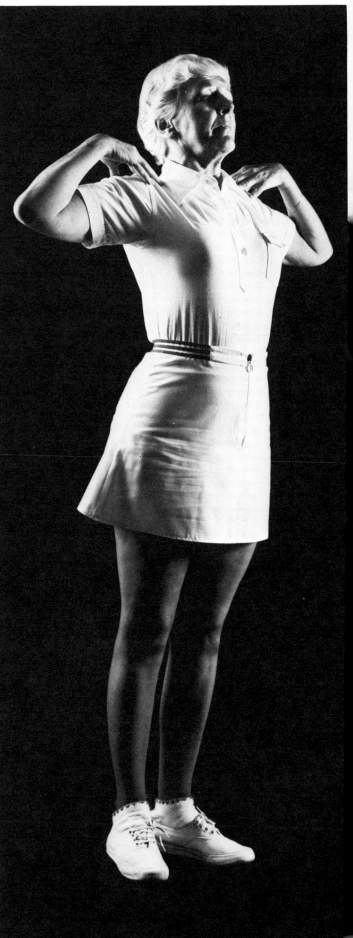

12 Breathing Exercise

- *Place your hands on your shoulders, keeping the back straight.*

- *Now breathe in, pulling your elbows back at the same time. Try to pull all the air from the room into your lungs.*

- *Breathe out in a long, forceful, sighing exhalation, at the same time bringing your elbows forward.*

- *When all the air is expelled, relax. Let your body sag like a rag doll.*

- *Then and only when you absolutely must, begin to inhale again.*

- *Do this at least five times. If you breathe too enthusiastically, you might feel a little dizzy. In that case, just cut down on the amount of air you push out.*

13 Neck Mobility Exercise

- *Put a book flat on your head.*
- *Now lean your body forward so that the book starts to fall, but adjust your neck to prevent the book from falling.*
- *Repeat this, twisting your body in all directions.*
- *You may hear some cracking and "clunking." Don't let that worry you. These are normal sounds; your head won't fall off!*
- *Three times (ten seconds each time) is enough to increase your flexibility with this exercise.*

14 Arm and Shoulder Strengthener

One of the best ways of increasing strength in the upper extremities is the push-up, but beware of the ordinary push-up from the floor. It can cause problems, because you lift your body weight when you do it. A less demanding exercise is the push-back from a wall. In this position the force of gravity is reduced.

This isotonic exercise is great for toning up your arms or shoulders.

- *Stand up straight facing the wall, your feet two steps back, with your arms at shoulder height, palms flat against the wall.*
- *Lean forward, with your hands still on the wall, and bend your elbows so that your nose touches the wall. Inhale as you lean forward, then push back and exhale.*
- *Let your heels lift from the ground as you lean forward and do it SLOWLY!*

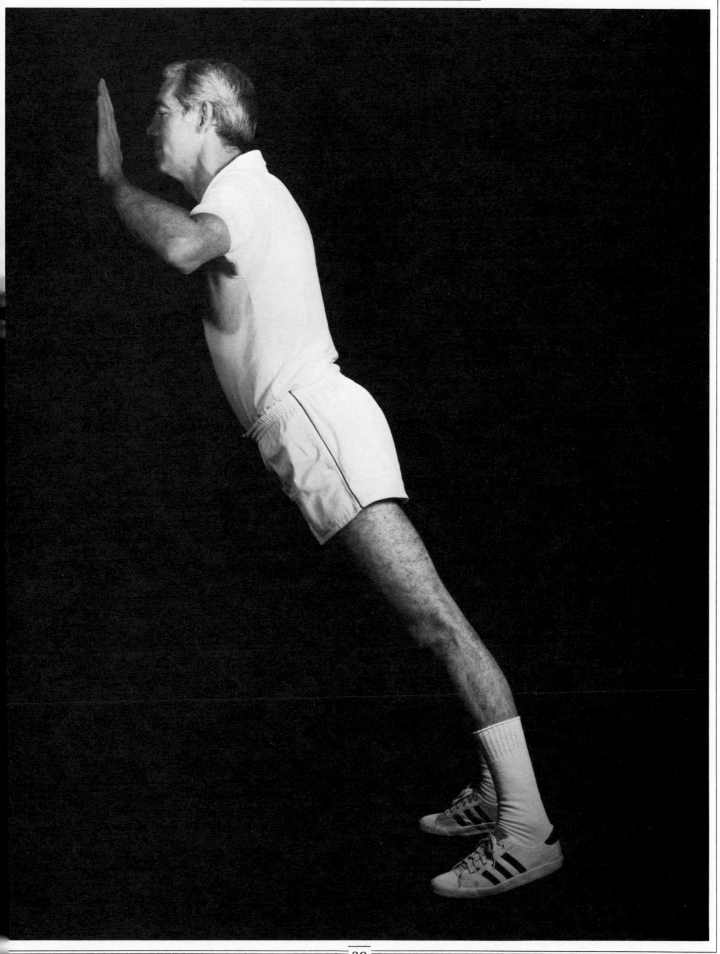

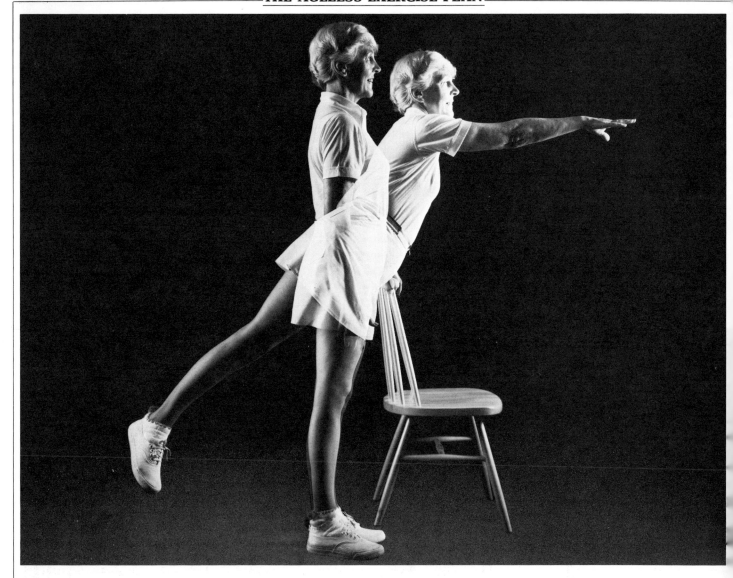

15 Lower Back and Buttocks Exercise

- *Stand straight beside your chair with your feet together.*
- *Place one hand on the back of the chair and hold the other in front at shoulder height. Lift one leg back and up, as far as possible keeping the knee straight.*
- *Now, return to the starting position and repeat with the other leg.*
- *You will feel this stretch on the upper front part of your thigh. Don't kick your heel up — just a nice, slow, steady pull which will increase your flexibility and give you a little more power.*
- *Do it three times with a bounce.*

16 Hip and Leg Exercise

- *Sit on the chair with your knees three inches apart.*
- *Put your fist between the knees and draw them together as tightly as you can for a count of three.*
- *Now relax the knees and move them apart, but prevent them from going apart by resisting with your hands on the outer sides of the knees.*
- *Press out for a count of three and then relax.*
- *Alternate this isometric movement five times.*

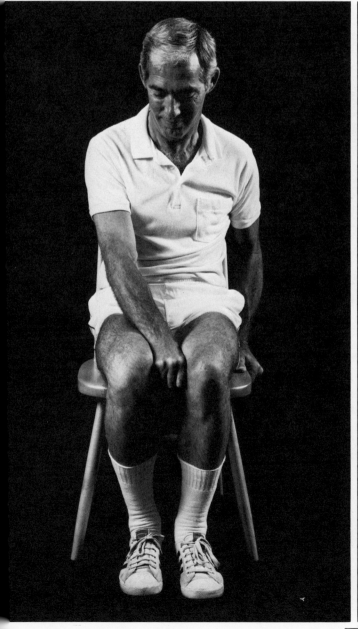
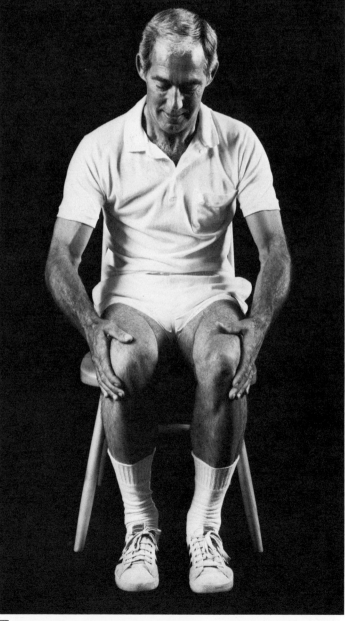

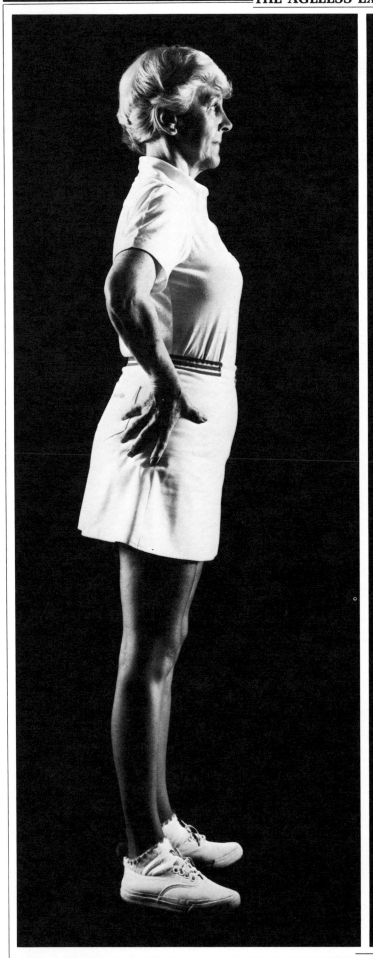
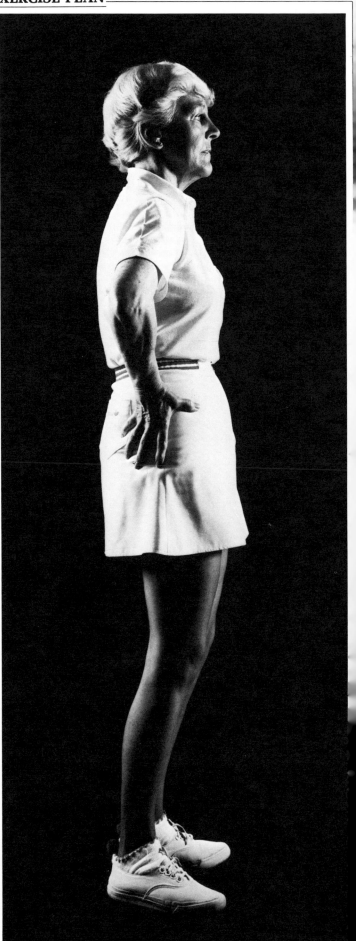

17 Pelvic Tilt

Standing straight and walking in comfort depend a great deal upon your abdominal muscles. You can tighten these by doing the following exercise.

- *Sit or stand. Pull your stomach in while inhaling and hold it for ninety seconds, then relax.*
- *The tilt part comes by rotating your pelvis backward, and tucking in your tail. Just imagine your pelvis is a dinner plate set at right angles to your hips. Now rotate those dinner plates front to back like a hula dancer. You'll feel the lower part of your back flatten and lose its curve.*
- *Then relax the tilt and your back will resume its normal position.*
- *Repeat this three times, to the count of three.*
- *Try keeping your pelvis tilted for as long as possible, before relaxing it again. Then walk around with the pelvis tilted and imagine someone is holding you up by your hair.*

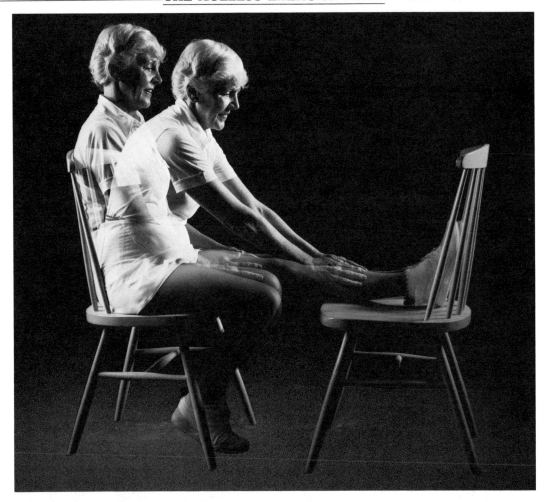

⇧ 18 Hamstring Stretching

Hamstring tightening is the most common cause of bad posture and chronic back pain.

- *To keep your hamstrings stretched, sit straight in your chair and put one leg on a chair opposite to you.*
- *Slowly bend forward from the waist feeling the pull in the back of the leg.*
- *Hold.*
- *Relax.*
- *Repeat with the other leg.*
- *Do this SLOWLY. Bounce this exercise a little so that you feel some tugging at the muscle.*

This movement is better than the usual attempts to touch your toes with your hands while standing. It should give you a "pull" feeling but not cause pain.

19 Ankle Exercise

Do you have problems clearing your toes from the steps as you go upstairs? How about strengthening your ankle muscles?

- *Sit straight in your chair with your feet planted on the floor in front of you.*
- *Now raise one foot as far as possible while keeping the heel on the floor by bending the ankle. That's easy.*
- *Now repeat it with the other foot but this time put the left foot on top and raise your right foot while pushing down with your left.*
- *Press down heavily enough to use effort to raise your right foot. The right side is contracting concentrically while the left resists.*
- *Alternate and do the same while stressing the left foot with the right. You need at least five isotonic lifts to build the necessary power.*

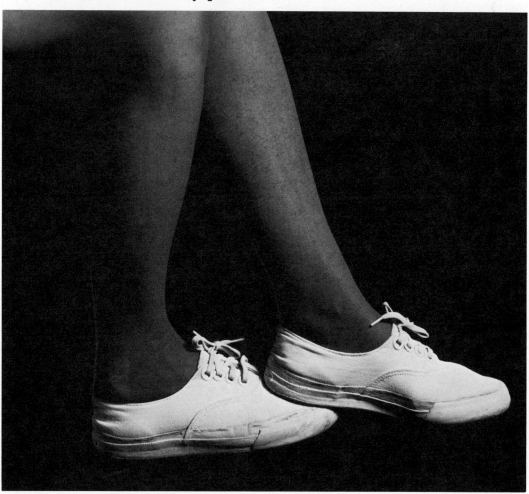

20 Hand Exercise

Keep your fingers mobile by stretching them as far as they will go.

- *Take the left index finger between your right index finger and thumb and press the left index finger back so that you are stretching the knuckle.*
- *Then go successively over each of the other fingers.*
- *Increase the strength of your grip by forming the fingers of one hand into a hook.*
- *Then form another hook with the opposite hand, hook the two hands together and try to pull them apart. Pull as hard as is comfortable with each hand.*

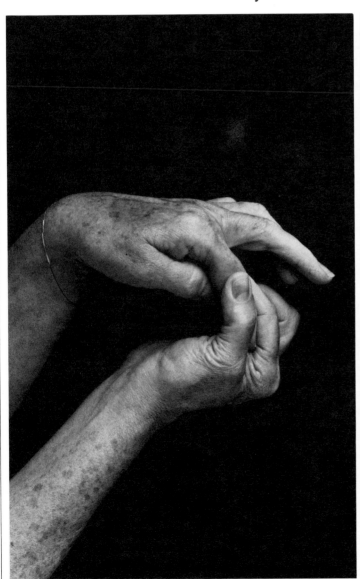
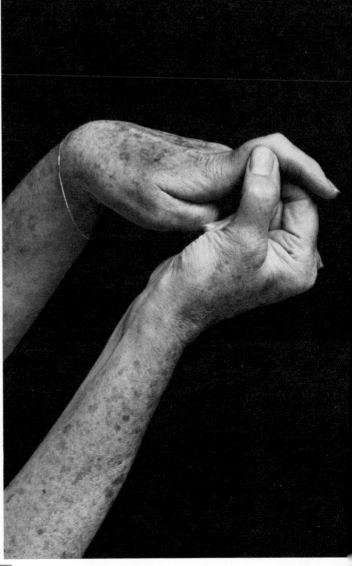

6
ADVANCED AGELESS EXERCISES

Like Oliver Twist, once you've developed an appetite for exercise, you will probably want "more." The exercises in this chapter provide extras for those who have successfully managed the Basic and Alternate Ageless Exercises. But don't forget. Always warm up and cool down after the sessions, no matter at what level you start. As well, make sure you do the breathing exercises outlined in the first section. They are a great start for any movement.

21 Neck Exercise

You have already done this exercise to maintain flexibility, which is part of the basis of fitness, page 24.

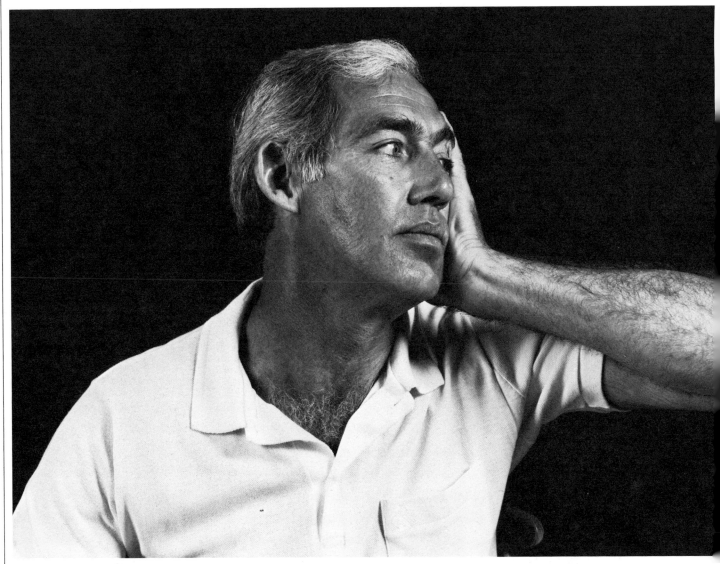

⇪ ◉ *Now repeat those movements, but this time press your left hand against the chin as you rotate your neck to the left and apply some resistance.*

◉ *Resist all the way as you turn the head from right to left.*

◉ *Repeat, this time moving it left to right.*

- *Lower your chin to the chest and then raise it so you face the ceiling.*
- *Look as far back as you can.*
- *Then bring your chin back to your chest.*
- *Do this rocking motion of the neck two times per session, and resist with one hand as shown in the photograph.*

This isotonic exercise gives the neck more stability by increasing the power of the muscles.

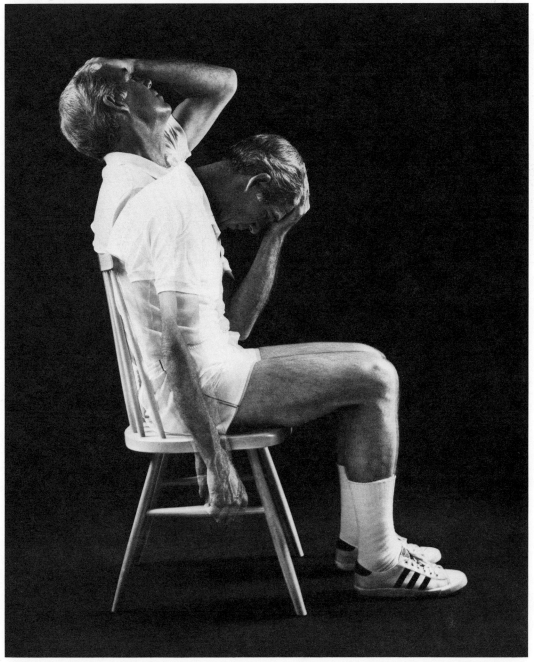

22 Side Stretch

- Raise the right arm to the ceiling beside your ear, curving gracefully like a ballerina.
- Let the left arm hang by your side.
- Take a deep breath, bend sideways and let the left arm slide slowly down your side.
- Bounce gently and push out your breath. Just feel how that stretches the right side of the body.
- Then take a deep breath in that position and go back to the upright position.
- Change to the left arm, exhaling, and repeat the movement on the other side.
- When you have gone as far as you can go, try a little extra bounce to give just one more pull.
- Do these flexibility exercises twice to each side alternately. Remember to take a deep breath before you bend and exhale completely while you are stretching as far as possible.

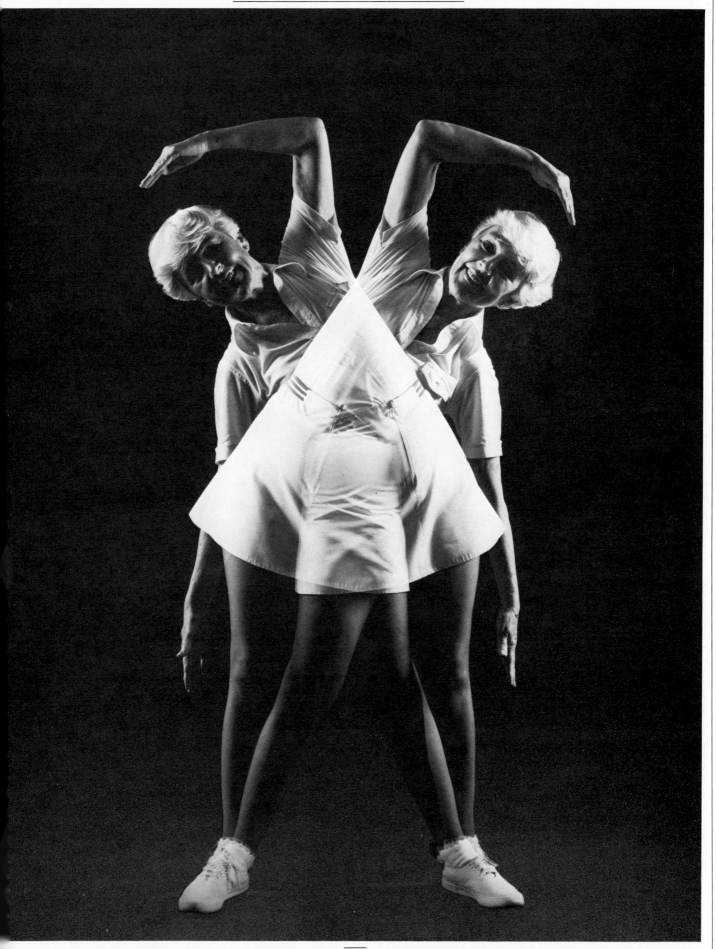

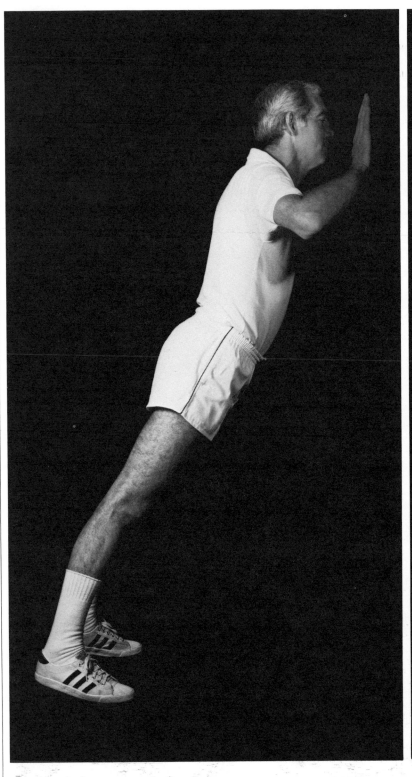
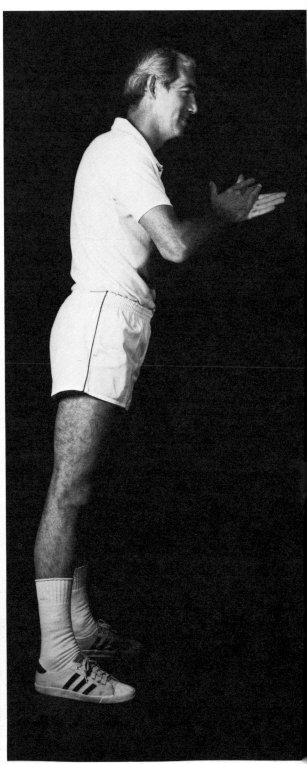

23 Feldman's Clapping Push-Back

This exercise combines both power building in the arms and shoulders and increased dexterity. Note that this is an eccentric exercise when your chin comes forward and a concentric one as you push back.

- *Stand facing the wall as you did when you were doing a push-back.*

- *Now let your body fall towards the wall to do the push-back, except when you return to the starting position, take your hands from the wall and clap, before your body falls forward again.*

- *It's a rhythmical movement as you sway forward and back.*

- *Inhale when leaning forward, exhale when returning to the start position. Do not make this a jerky movement. It should be a smooth, continuous action and it should be possible to clap six times before your body comes back to the wall.*

- *Do it for two minutes.*

24 Sit-Ups

Sit-ups are exercises for building super stomach muscles.

- *Lie on your back with your knees bent and feet flat on the floor.*

- *Secure your feet under a piece of furniture or a strap or have someone hold your feet to prevent them from raising during the "sit-up."*

- *Now place your hands across your stomach with your elbows clear of the floor.*

- *Raise your torso to an upright position and try to touch your forehead to your knees.*

- *Exhale as you come up and inhale as you curl back down to the starting position. Try to do this slowly so that you are not jerking as you start to go up. Imagine you are wearing a belt. It should be the last thing to leave the floor as you come up and the first thing to touch it on the return to the starting position. (This is a concentric exercise, but you can also do it eccentrically if you sit back after sitting up.)*

- *When you can do this as easily as a summer breeze, try it with your hands on your chest, and then behind your neck and finally, stretched straight out over your head.*

- *If you can do this five times as an advanced exercise, there is a guarantee that you will have a stomach like an ironing board.*

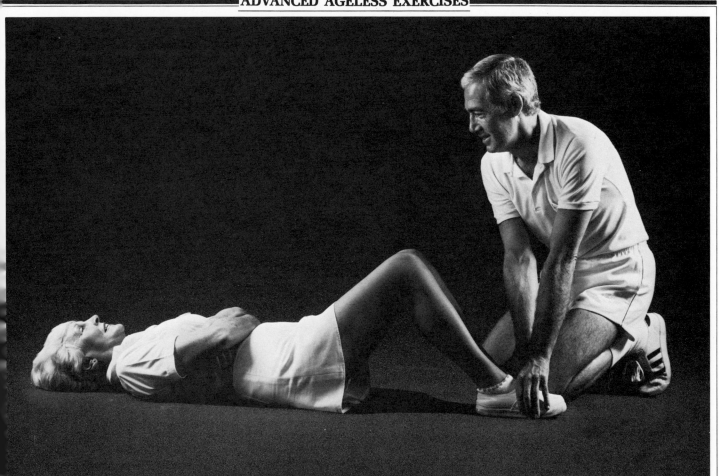

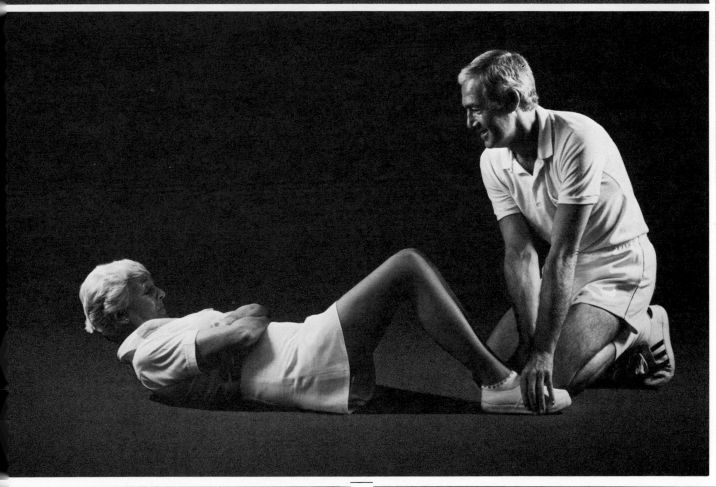

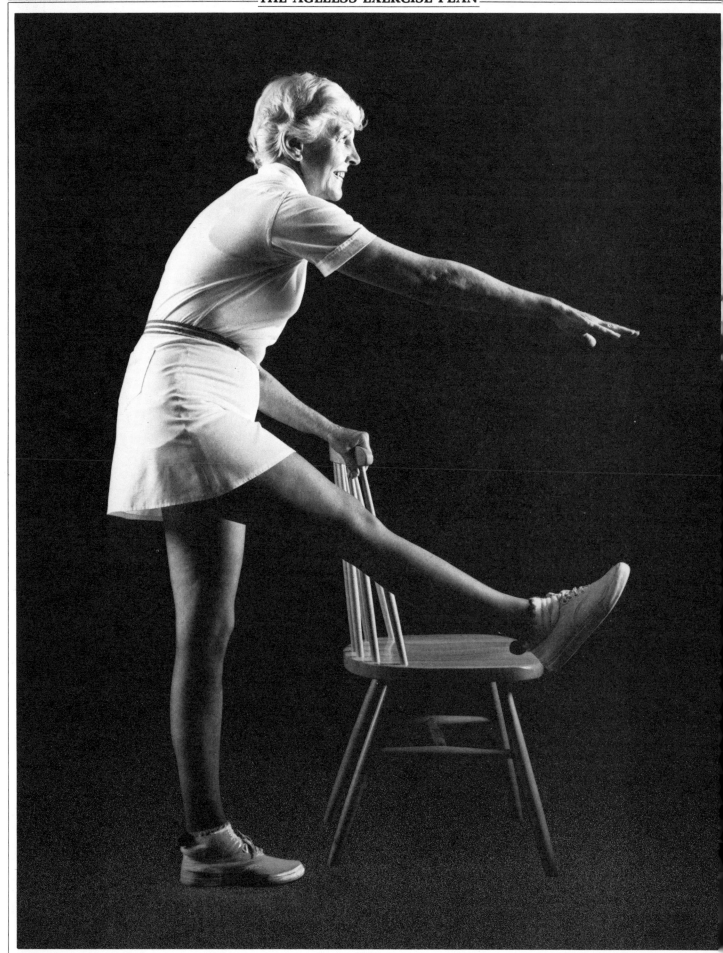

25 The Hamstring Kick

- *Stand up straight with one hand on the back of a chair.*
- *Raise your free hand to waist level directly in front of your body and then slowly kick your leg up to meet your hand. You'll feel a pull in the upper back part of your leg.*
- *Return to the starting position and repeat on the opposite side.*
- *Next place your hand at chest level and repeat slowly.*
- *When you do the "kick" do it gently, not as though you were trying to boot a ball sixty yards, but rather as in a slow-motion dance.*
- *Three times is enough to prevent your hamstrings from shrinking and to maintain good posture and avoid back strain.*

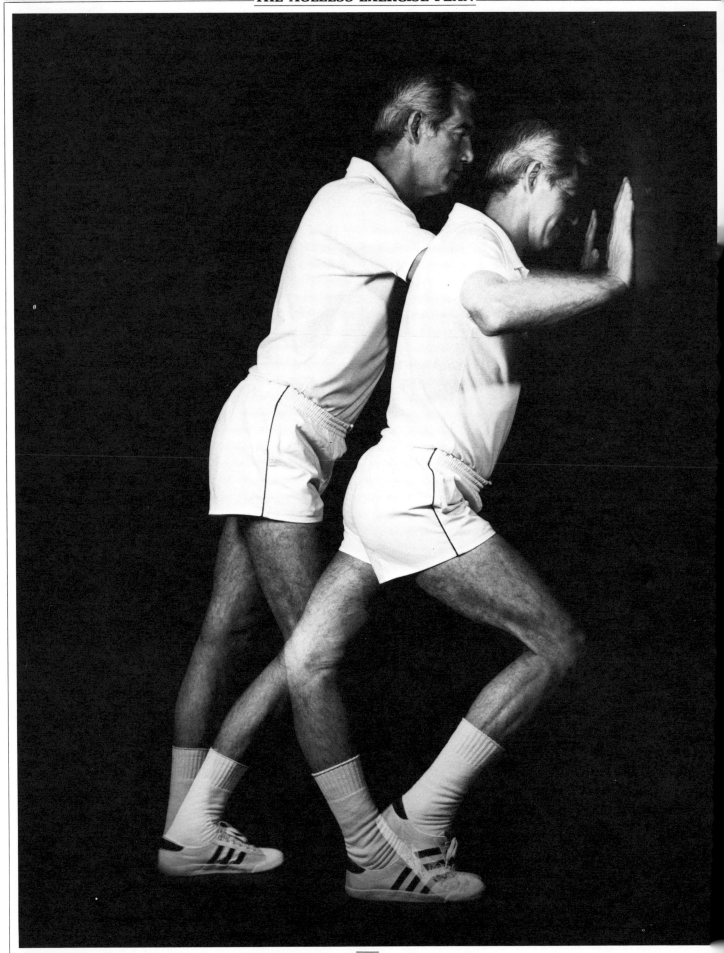

26 Calf Stretch

While you are doing the kick, you'd better make sure that the calf muscles in the back of the leg are not tightening with this exercise.

- *Stand straight with your hands extended at shoulder level, palms touching the wall.*
- *Step back two foot lengths, leaning forward against the wall with your hands. Be sure your feet are flat on the floor.*
- *Now flex one knee and lean forward on your bent leg and you will feel the pull in the bottom of the opposite straight leg in the calf region.*
- *Don't bounce this one, just stretch out slowly for five times and then change leg positions.*

27 Calf Raise

This isotonic toe-raising develops your calf muscles and takes the pain out of stair climbing.

- *Stand behind your chair, with your feet nine inches apart, and then SLOWLY raise your body up on one foot lifting the heel.*
- *Stay up as long as you can, using the chair to keep your balance.*
- *Now return to the starting position.*
- *Do it five times on each foot.*

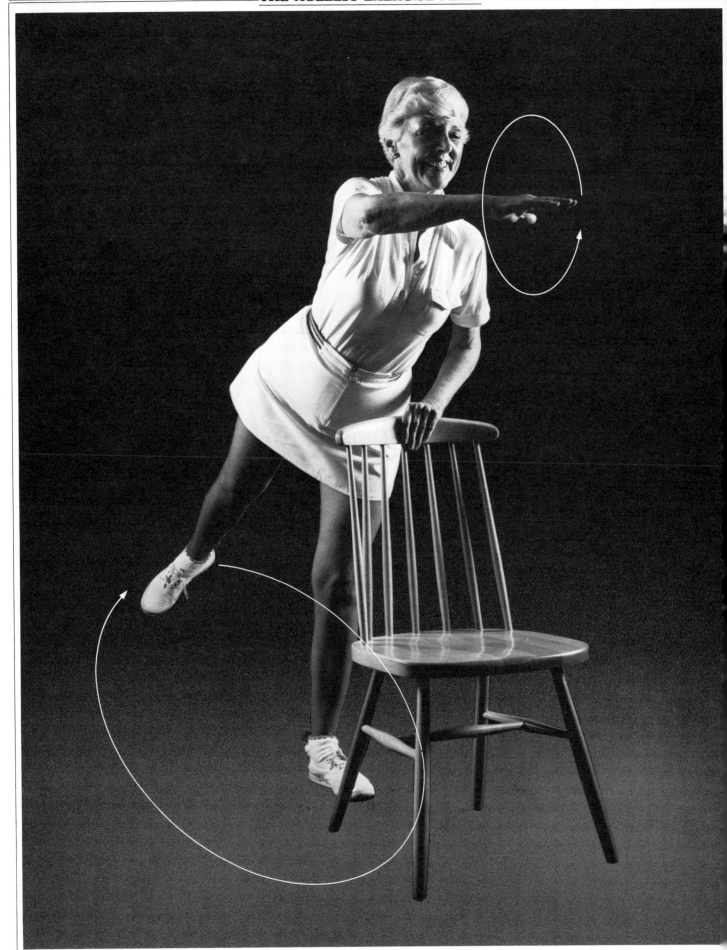

28 Leg and Arm Swings

How about something a little more energetic? There's nothing like this one for stirring the blood!

- *Stand by your chair, keeping your arm close to the chair for support.*
- *Slowly start swinging your free arm forward in a circle and leg backwards in a circle in the opposite direction.*
- *Increase the speed gradually until you are out of breath.*
- *Now stop.*
- *Repeat the exercise with the other arm and leg.*

29 Hand Exercise

Having trouble opening jars?

- *Squeeze a handball as directed previously but now throw it gently up and clap your hands before catching it.*
- *Relax and do the same with your left hand.*
- *Repeat this same action but this time throw the ball a little higher and clap twice before you catch it.*
- *Continue and you will be able to clap four times before catching the ball again.*

It's great, not only for strengthening, but for the coordination which you need for hand tasks.

30 Facial Muscles

Most people forget to stimulate the tone of the muscles which are important for "special" actions — such as communicating or just plain looking beautiful. The face has many more small, specific muscles than any other part of the body. As with the other exercises, begin the facial program by relaxation.

- *Tap your face with your fingertips, first your forehead then your cheeks, then your chin and neck.*
- *Tap each muscle deliberately, letting it relax and sag and then tighten it up as much as you can.*
- *Screw your face up.*
- *Then go to each area, tap and relax and tighten.*
- *Then give your skin a good rub with the tip of your thumb to bring more color into it and cause the muscles to tighten.*
- *Now contract your forehead or your cheek or chin muscles and resist the movements with your finger.*
- *Contract the muscles as firmly as you can and resist as strongly as possible without bruising the skin.*
- *Do these isometric exercises in front of a mirror each morning and night for the best results.*

7
THE PROBLEM EXERCISER

Why is it that some over-fifties fail to get into an exercise program? Commonly it's because they have a health problem. This may range from a minor disability to serious disease such as heart trouble. But, in fact, there is no reason why you cannot reach a higher level of fitness even though some disorder has been diagnosed and treatment is being received. If that's the case, this chapter contains special exercises for you.

31 Heart Disorder

If you do have a heart problem, it makes sense to ask your doctor just what exercises you can do. Although your pulse rate may be normal when you are doing simple exercises, when heavier effort drives the beats up to 160 per minute, there could be some harmful irregularities especially if you have hypertension.

So, to repeat, have a medical check-up before beginning the Ageless Exercise Plan. If there is a problem, your doctor can test you on an exercise bicycle. You pedal against a known load for a specific length of time while an electrocardiogram is taken to determine where you are on the physical fitness scale. After the test you will be told what limits should be put on the amount of activity attempted every day.

But having a heart disorder should not deter you. It is well accepted by the medical profession that people with coronary problems should exercise to increase the level of their heart function and to raise their general scale of well-being. If your other muscles are stronger, then there is less demand on your ticker.

In older people, a common problem is congestive heart disease: the heart has difficulty handling the circulation, blood becomes pooled in the legs, and swelling develops around the ankles. This edema, which can also be felt in the lower part of the back or in the abdomen, not only slows you down and gives you shortness of breath, but may also lead to some skin breakdown. So when you are exercising with swollen ankles, be sure not to scrape or break the skin, or put a great deal of pressure on your legs. For example, all crossed-leg types of exercises should be avoided. It's necessary to grade your efforts carefully to avoid too much demand on the circulatory system. Generally isotonic exercises are better than isometric as they do not elevate the blood pressure.

Hardening of the arteries is another circulation problem that may affect your exercises. This disorder, called peripheral vascular disease, results in your arms and legs being starved for blood. They usually feel cold and look pale. Those heavy socks aren't necessary because it's cold outside; it's cold inside! This coldness may be accompanied by a burning and a numb-type of pain in the feet. There are no specific exercises to persuade the arteries to open up allowing a normal flow. However, lifting your feet and then dropping them to the floor level can be of some help.

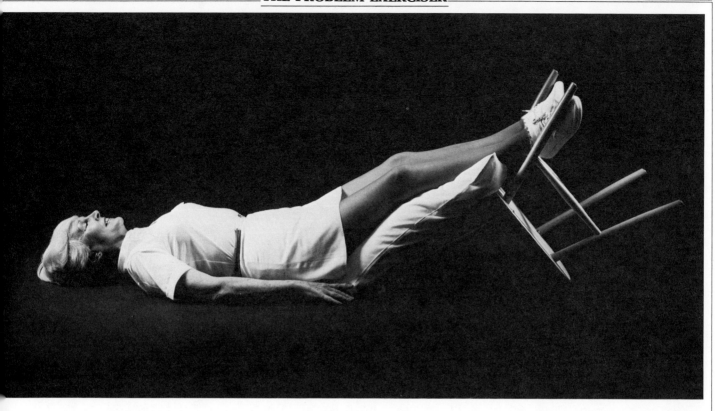

⇧ **31**

- *Lie in bed with your legs elevated above the heart level for thirty seconds and then drop them below that level for fifteen seconds.*
- *Put your feet up on the back of a chair which has been turned upside down on the mattress.*
- *Always start with the legs up and work through the sequence up/down three times, finishing with the legs up again.*

This exercise promotes an increased ebb and flow of blood and may aid in clearing away the end products of muscle contractions and in bringing freshly oxygenated blood to the feet.

When doing any general exercises with impaired circulation, do short bursts of activity, up to three minutes long. Then rest and begin another burst after two minutes. This gives the reduced blood flow a chance to restore the energy cells of the muscles by bringing in new supplies of oxygen.

32/33/34 Poor Balance

You'll notice when exercising, how important it is to have good balance. Certainly you can't do standing, unsupported exercise unless your feet are well placed on the ground and your balance is secure. Try pirouetting without a good sense of balance and you'll end up on the floor!

Poor balance is common in older people, which is the reason they may walk slower with the feet farther apart than when they were young. This decreased ability to maintain balance shows itself particularly when walking. Try to cross the floor slowly and observe that for one-third of the time during the step you have to maintain equilibrium on one leg. This requires a great deal of muscle power. One-legged exercises can be very helpful.

32

- *Stand between two dining-room chairs with your hands poised just above their backs.*
- *Now take the left foot from the floor and stand on the right foot for five seconds.*
- *Then stand with the left foot on the floor with your right foot in the air. Notice that you will begin to sway towards the end of the time allotment and will need to hold the chairs.*
- *This exercise should be done at least ten times on each foot each day.*
- *Next do the same exercise, only stand on the toes of one foot, and then the other.*
- *The last movement to fully develop your balance muscles is to stand up on your heel alone.*

After a while you will notice as you walk, that during the time your weight is on one foot, your ability to maintain yourself in an upright position is improving. Your speed will increase and your step will be more certain. If you are unable to regain all your sense of balance, then a cane in either hand will enable you to walk for miles — and is also useful to control yapping dogs!

However, this inability to maintain normal balance may be due to a number of other causes. For example, if there's something wrong with your peripheral nervous system — as may happen with low grade diabetes — and you're not getting the sensory signals back from the feet, and there's some uncertainty about where your feet are on the ground, then the following simple exercises should be done.

33

- ◉ *Walk backwards.*
- ◉ *Do it slowly and deliberately, touching the ground first with the forefoot, then the whole sole and last lifting your toes off, so only the heel is in contact.*
- ◉ *Now do it faster. It's excellent for your equilibrium!*
- ◉ *Next, attempt to rely only on the sensations from your feet and walk with your eyes closed. This is good for developing increased sensors in your toes.*

On the other hand, your balance mechanism may be upset because of a middle ear disorder. Infection in the middle ear, labyrinthitis, is a common problem and is often associated with a viral attack. The middle ear is like a finely built watch — a highly complicated balance organism. It can be knocked out of order by various infections. When it is involved, you will notice there is difficulty in rising from sitting to standing or in changing the position of your head. For example, you may hear a horn blast on the road, turn your head to see what's going on, and immediately have a swimming sensation when all the world seems to be going around. This can last for only a second or two, but it can be very disconcerting.

Some people carry a knotted handkerchief in their pocket, because it helps to have something to hold onto when the dizzy episode occurs. Alternatively, you can grab onto a lamppost or piece of furniture to steady yourself. The typical stance during a dizzy episode is with the feet wide apart, as though you were on a ship expecting it to dive and roll.

Indeed the ship analogy is a good one because sometimes there is a little nausea. The treatment for labyrinthitis is a medical one and requires medication such as anti-seasickness pills. But what about exercises?

34

- *Sit in a swivel chair and turn slowly to accustom those middle ear sensors to some movements.*

- *Build up your tolerance to moving rapidly. Go through a greater range of movement in slow stages, by rotating the chair with your feet. Once again, do this exercise with your eyes open and closed.*

While doing other exercises, if you do experience dizziness, put yourself in a position where there is no danger of falling. Contrary to the general instructions, most exercises should be done while seated in an armchair, particularly when the activity involves movement of the head. However, if sitting in a chair or even lying in a bed is not secure enough a position to prevent you from feeling considerable distress when the episodes come, it is absolutely vital that you see your family physician for a medication to help you gain more control.

Of course, you may be having difficulties with your balance simply because the muscles in your legs are not strong enough. If so, then exercises 16, 18 and 19 for strengthening the muscles in the legs are appropriate. In addition to these, you should do some of the advanced exercises: 25, 26, 27 or 28.

35/36 Post-mastectomy

There are a number of conditions which, having received

medical treatment, still deter people from getting back into a normal exercise program. Amputation of the breast for cancer is one example. After a mastectomy operation, you require an exercise plan for the shoulder, elbow and wrist of the affected side, as it is vital to maintain a full range of movement in all these joints. Do this exercise.

35

⦿ *Put the hand of the operated side behind your neck slowly, with the arm at shoulder level and draw the elbow back as far behind you as possible and then as far forward as possible.*

⦿ *Then reach with the hand of the affected side down to the lower part of the back and raise your fingers up between the shoulder blades.*

⦿ *Take a towel with the normal hand, drop it behind the shoulders and use it to pull the other hand up to the shoulder blades.*

⦿ *This is a stretching exercise for the shoulder and should be done three times per day.*

The stiffening that occurs post-operatively can be prevented by this routine of maintaining flexibility of the shoulder joint.

Post-mastectomy lymphoedema, where there is a massive swelling of the arm, can become inflamed and painful and, in some cases, dangerous to your health. Edema is usually caused by obstruction to the return of lymph into the normal bloodstream. This obstruction can be the result of fibrosis following the operation or x-radiation for the treatment of cancer. Most women establish a nice balance between the normal flow and the obstruction so that although there may be a little swelling in the arm, it never becomes grossly distended. Nevertheless, through over-activity the balance of circulation is sometimes upset leading to massive swelling — lymphoedema. If this occurs, it is necessary to do a specific set of exercises for the involved arm.

36

⊛ *Wind an elastic bandage (Ace⊤) around your arm, from hand to shoulder, while it is elevated, and then make a fist slowly.*

⊛ *Repeat this twenty times.*

The increased pressure generated inside the forearm by the muscle bulging against the elastic bandage will help to drive the fluid out of the arm. The remainder of the shoulder and general exercises may be done in the normal fashion.

37 Arthritis

Arthritis may present some difficulties to the would-be exerciser. There are two major types of joint disease. One, rheumatoid arthritis, is associated with deformity of the body; the fingers, knees and feet may be quite abnormal. The other, more common type, is osteoarthritis, which affects many in the over-fifties' group and is not usually seen with any deformity aside from nodules on the fingers. Areas of osteoarthritis in the neck, lumbar region, knees and shoulders can cause restrictions of movement while exercising. Sometimes the joints clunk and squeak like an old rusty garden-gate. It's up to you to prevent that rust from forming!

The Ageless Exercise Plan stresses that it is necessary to increase your range of movement and maintain flexibility in the neck and back. This applies particularly to persons with osteoarthritis, who usually have stiffness in the morning and difficulty in moving about after a long session of sitting. The joints tend to freeze up.

If there is some osteoarthritis in your neck, which may be accompanied by disc trouble, the normal rotation-type exercises, 2 and 13, should not be done while standing. Rather, lie flat on your bed with your head on a pillow.

37

- *Rotate your neck to the right as far as it will go and then slowly rotate your neck to the left, also as far as it will go.*
- *Do this flexibility routine three times a session, trying to get a little more movement at the end of each turn.*
- *To do this, put your finger on your chin, when your head is fully turned to the right and give a very gentle, even push to the chin in order to get one or two more degrees of movement.*
- *Then rotate to the left and do the same pushing tactic. These exercises differ from the previous inasmuch as you are pushing for an increase of ten degrees of movement.*
- *Now with your left hand on your forehead, try to bring your head forward from the pillow but prevent it with your hand. This is an isometric exercise and is designed to strengthen the muscles alongside the neck.*
- *Next, while flat on your back with your face looking directly at the ceiling, put your right hand on your right cheek and tighten the neck muscles trying to rotate your head to the right.*
- *Resist with the right hand. This is another isometric exercise, but this one is exercising the rotators of the neck.*
- *Do the same exercise on the left.*
- *Do each of these three times to a count of three.*

38/39 Back Pain

Low back pain seems to be epidemic in any age group, but it can be quite disabling, particularly when you are in your forties and fifties. Most of the time it is caused by chronic strain to the joints of the spine, which results largely from changes in posture and an increase in abdominal obesity. Chapters 4 and 5 talked about how to control what is going on in your midsection. The exercises in those chapters are also important for the lumbar spine.

The back is a series of bones, vertebrae, shaped like building blocks, and linked to one another by a system of short and long ligaments and muscles. The short ones connect each bone to the adjacent one. The long ones span several of the bones. A problem can occur when one or more of these muscles become weakened through inactivity or chronic stretching. Such chronic stretching often takes place when you stand and allow your stomach to bulge forward, like an alderman at a flower show. You can prevent looking like him by doing some special back exercises.

But first let's look at the spine in its entirety. Each of the building block bones can be joined into a solid bony structure by the action of short muscles and ligaments, like putting a snake into a freezer. The fluid flexibility is replaced by a rigid rod. This overall control of the whole back is maintained by a series of longer muscles, which holds the back straight in the same way a flagpole is held erect by guy wires. There are guy wires in the front of the abdomen, in the back and on each side.

The guy wires in back, the extensor muscles, are usually well developed because they are the ones that hold you erect whenever you stand. However, the guy wires in the front, called abdominal or flexor muscles, are frequently not well maintained and when they are weak, the flagpole starts to buckle. To compensate for this, the extensor muscles out-pull the flexors, causing you to lean backwards, which leads to a chronic strain of the joints between the vertebrae.

To maintain those anterior guys or abdominal muscles you must do sit-up exercise 24. However, here is a special type of sit-up exercise for those of you with back pain. Doing a sit-up in the normal manner causes a considerable increase of pressure on the discs, which are the shock absorbers between the vertebrae in the lower part of your back. That pressure can be handled easily by the normal spine. But with some of the changes in the discs and surrounding vertebrae that may accompany osteoarthritis, it is better to avoid this high pressure by doing a sit-back, rather than a sit-up.

38

- *A sit-back is an eccentric-type exercise. Start it while you are in bed or on the floor.*
- *Bend your knees and put your feet flat on the floor under a bureau or a strap, or have someone hold them down.*

- *Now, while seated put your hands around your knees.*

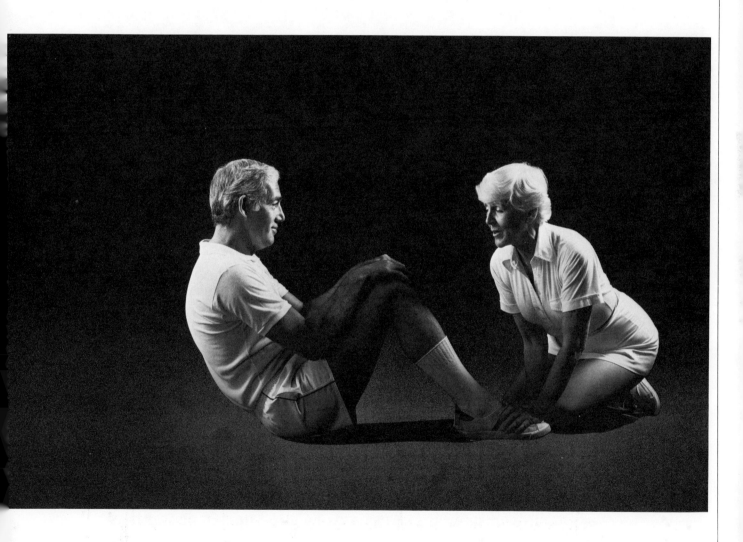

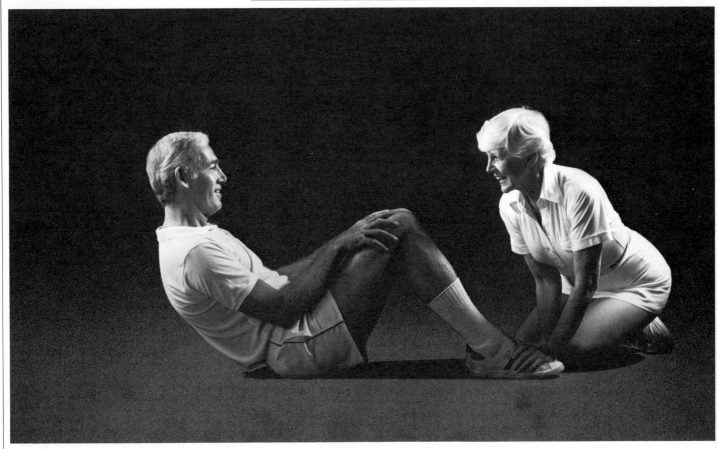

 ● Let yourself fall slowly back onto the floor using your hands on your legs to control the speed so that you do not over-exert your abdominal muscles. Can you feel them tighten up as you sit back?

● When you are fully relaxed on the floor, begin to come up to your first position, that is with your hands on your knees. However, don't curl yourself up as you do in a sit-up. Rather crawl up sideways, using your legs as a support and pulling yourself up with your hands and elbows.

● Repeat this sit-back procedure and notice that as you do so the abdominal muscles tighten and you get a feeling of pressure under whatever is holding your feet flat on the floor.

This sit-back exercise takes care of a good deal of abdominal weakness. When you are able to do it fairly easily, but still have some weakness of the abdominals, then you can begin doing some of the concentric-type sit-ups. But it's not necessary to do a full sit-up.

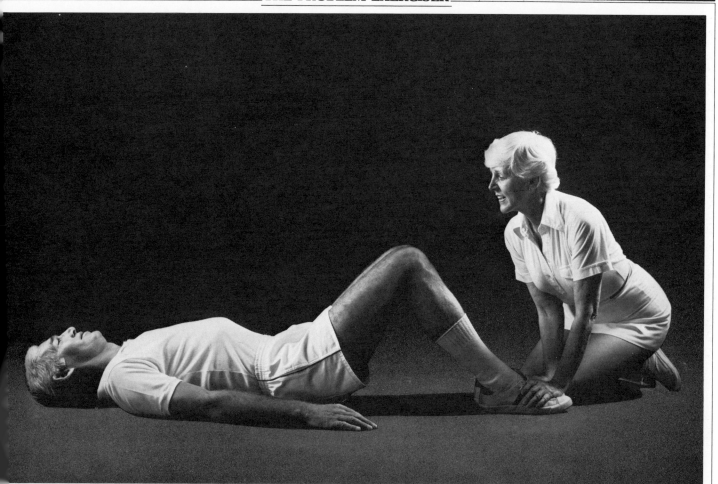

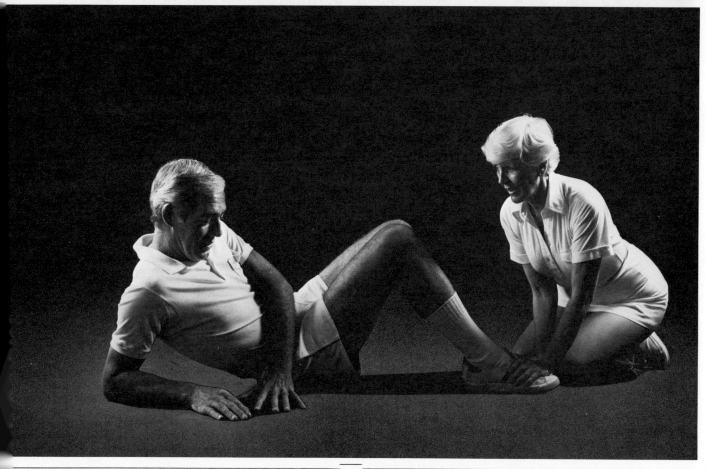

39

- *With your back flat on the floor, your knees flexed, and your feet held down, begin to sit up reaching with your hands for your knees.*
- *But don't come up all the way, just clear the floor with your shoulders and then drop back. This will make an angle of about fifteen degrees between your trunk and the floor.*
- *Do this to the count of three, that is up/up/up, hold/hold/hold, back/back/back, relax/relax/relax.*

This exercise builds power and can be done progressively. Start with three each morning and evening and increase slowly to fifteen.

40/41 Knee Problems

You read earlier about exercises for the quadriceps, the key muscle that stabilizes the knee joint. These are valuable especially after you've had a spell of enforced bed rest or if you have osteoarthritis of the knee, which may show itself by stiffness and pain in the morning or after a long walk. To build up the quadriceps and stabilize the knee, you should do exercises 9, 16 and 25 and the ones below.

One quandary in exercising with weak knee muscles is a tendency for the tibia, the lower leg bone, to fall back on the thigh bone, with the result that the knee is no longer perfectly aligned.

40

- *To overcome this, lie on your chest.*
- *Now bend the knees to make a ninety-degree angle with the floor. You are now about to exercise the right quadricep.*

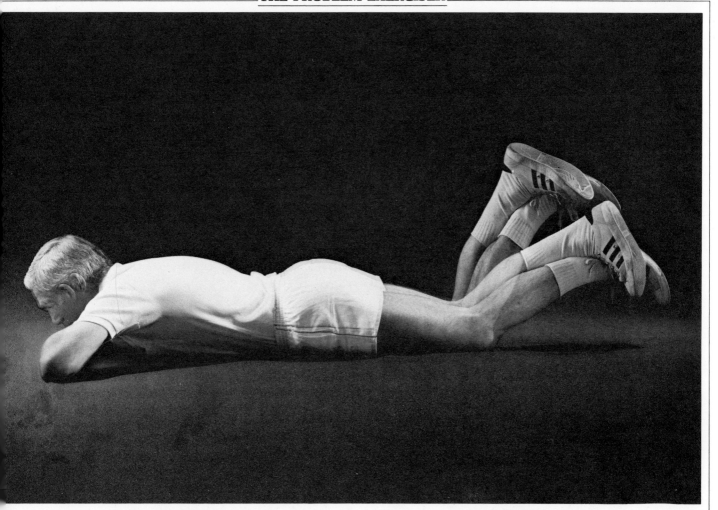

⇧ ⦿ *Straighten the right leg, that is extend the knee so the foot comes down to the floor. However, prevent the foot from reaching the floor by putting your left heel in front of the right tibia.*

⦿ *Press down with the right tibia, press up with the left heel, but do not stop the movement. Just resist with the left so that the right quadricep must work a little harder in order to get the leg out straight; i.e., toes to the floor.*

⦿ *Do this five times using the three count to pace yourself.*

⦿ *Then reverse the procedure and extend the left knee with resistance by the right foot and ankle.*

This is an isotonic concentric exercise for the quadriceps on one leg and an eccentric one for the other!

Another excellent way to build up your quadriceps is in the swimming pool.

41

⊙ *Stand in the water at waist level and do deep knee bends. The water will give buoyancy and will protect you from being overenthusiastic.*

Wearing flippers can give more resistance and increase the demand on the muscle. Doing deep knee bends on land can sometimes be a little dangerous as it tends to put undue stress on the cartilages about the knee, but the exercise can be done between two dining-room chairs with the backs turned to you. This provides the opportunity to reduce the strain on the joints and lets you recover your balance if you pitch forwards or backwards. You can do deep knee bends while standing on the toes or with the feet flat on the floor. Try both and note the different muscles which are pulled; each of these exercises uses a different group of muscles in your legs. Both are necessary.

42/43 Osteoporosis

One out of four women over forty suffers from loss of calcium in the bones, leading to a brittle bone type of condition called osteoporosis. The bones can no longer handle heavy loading and may crumble like an eggshell. Some have this condition without realizing its presence. It may become apparent for the first time when an extreme pain on trying to raise a window signals that there has been a minor collapse of one of the vertebrae in the back. Now this doesn't cause paralysis or impair muscle function, but it can be quite painful.

Although the condition of osteoporosis is treated by medication, its prevention can be promoted by exercise. Actually, basic exercises of the isotonic type will increase bone calcium content, and even local exercises to a specific joint will result in firmer bones in that one area. If you examine an old tennis player, she has firmer bones in her raquet arm compared with the less active arm.

The most common place for osteoporosis is in the spine. Here is a set of special exercises to treat that area specifically. This program recognizes that when the trunk is bent forward there is a tendency to compress each vertebra along its front edge. If there is some loss of bone calcium, pressure is placed on the forward portion of the vertebra and it collapses slightly, turning its rectangular shape into a wedge shape. Like an eggshell it doesn't break; it tends to collapse. A humpback and loss of height are signs of this condition.

Those who have a tendency towards osteoporosis should avoid flexion exercises of the isometric type. Instead, do an extension isotonic one.

42

⬇

- *While lying on your stomach, extend the head and neck as though you were going to arise from the prone position. You'll feel the muscles in your back tighten when you do this. This exercise can be augmented, after you can do it easily, by putting the hands behind the back and moving as though diving up into the air.*

- *This type of exercise should be done to the count of three, five times.*

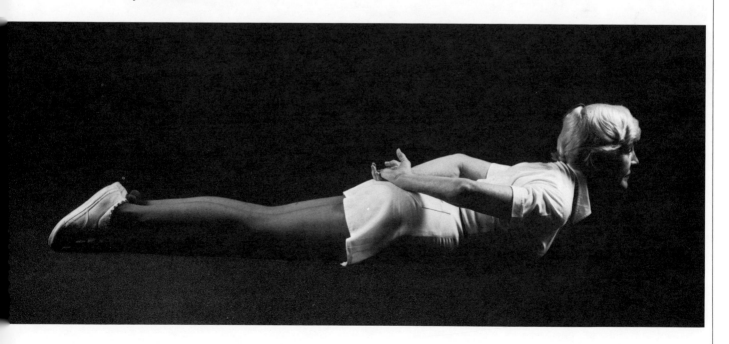

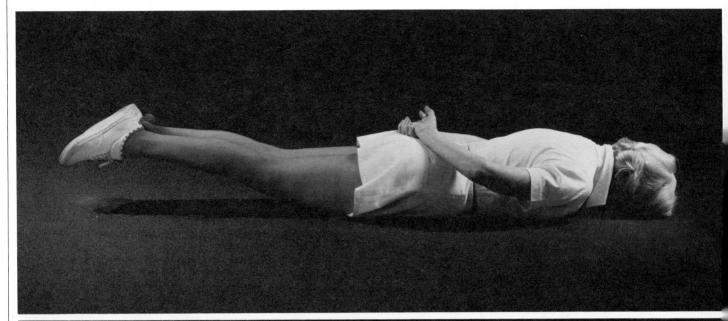

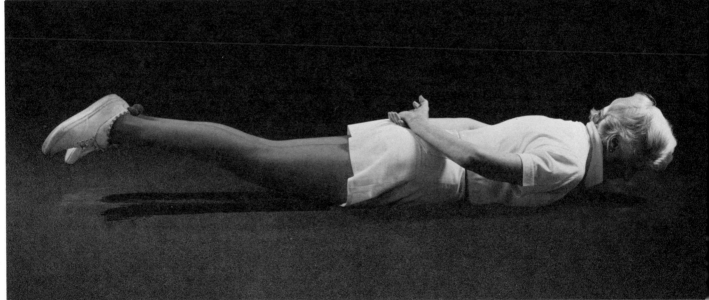

⇑ ◉ Then reverse and raise the legs rather than your head and neck. This extends the lower part of the lumbar spine.

◉ Finally, when you're very, very good at this particular exercise, you can do both movements together and turn your body into a rocker.

But, be careful! Although this exercise treats the osteoporotic portion of the back, it may aggravate other problems such as an arthritis or disc problem in the neck or lumbar spine. Both of these conditions are made worse by extension exercises. Other exercises in the Ageless Exercise Plan which will help the person with osteoporosis are 4, 14, 17, 22 and 23.

How do you manage when you have two problems at the same time? Carefully. Do the extension exercises isometrically without raising your head or feet from the floor. Just tighten up the muscles and start to go into the extension phase, but don't take it any further than that. Swimming or exercising in the pool is excellent for the osteoporotic back.

Of course, just because there is osteoporosis, it doesn't mean that the other reasons for flexibility can be forgotten.

43

◉ *To maintain forward flexibility of the trunk, it's necessary to bend over only while in a chair and try to touch the toes.*

◉ *Keep the motion forward in a straight line and avoid twisting the trunk as you do it the necessary three times per day.*

Diabetes

The diabetic may worry that a fitness program may upset his or her insulin requirements and cause blood glucose level abnormalities. It is true that the three-point control of diabetes — calorie intake, energy expenditure or exercise, and insulin — is usually in fine balance, and irregular high energy expenditures through sporadic exercising can cause difficulties. But a regular exercise regimen which builds up slowly allows for compensation of the other two factors and in the end leads to a significant decrease in the need for insulin. In addition, the circulation may be improved, reducing some of the threat of vascular complications, due to better control of cholesterol. If, however, you are a "brittle" diabetic, it is better to have a specific exercise program prescribed by your physician.

There is a problem in exercising when you have some other medical condition which may contraindicate that particular activity. But by working carefully, and figuring out which exercises do not cause pain, you can proceed sanely towards your goal of physical fitness. The main object of performing the exercises described in this chapter is to maintain mobility. Usually the development of muscle power is a secondary feature. It's better to be flexible and able to roll with the punches of modern living than to have bulging biceps.

8
LIFESTYLE
ACTIVITIES

Calisthenic exercises should be only a part of any program. Some people get a charge from them, but others find it difficult to maintain a constant level.

That's why it's necessary for you to be on a year-round planned program which will alternate your exercises and take advantage of the fitness that results from lifestyle activities. So in addition to the specific physical activities that have been outlined in this book, you have to begin thinking fitness. To join the fit after fifty brigade, start planning now on an activity program that is fun, makes living interesting and can be done for the rest of your long, long life.

With this extension of the general exercise plan, you can burn up more calories and can eat more heartily. Just think, with an exercise program you can eat cake without guilt! All you need to do is to make sure that your level of fitness consciousness is raised, and you avoid doing things the effortless way. If it's two flights of stairs, walk up! Don't take the elevator. If it's less than six flights of stairs, walk down. Escalators? No, unless you're carrying parcels. Want a lift? No, thanks, I'm walking.

The key to this lifestyle approach is an increase in your

everyday activity. A little rain shouldn't keep you under the bed covers. Make up your exercise plan to get around nature's little quirks. Indoor exercise activities, in addition to the general program, can use some simple pieces of equipment which will raise your energy fitness without lowering your bank account too much.

An exercise cycle is a helpful gadget. Buy a good one that will stand up through years of pedaling. Make sure that there is an adjustable screw so that you can put more resistance on the pedals and grade your activities. It should have a speedo-meter so that you can measure your output constantly. Most exercycles need simple maintenance such as you'd give to an ordinary bike, but in particular, make sure the resistance rollers which are applied to the wheel are trued up to prevent uneven wear on the wheel. You can even alter your exercycle so that you can read while cycling — just attach a board to the handle-bars and away you go.

Another indoor helper is a step-box. Take a sturdy wooden box, which is half the height between your knee and the floor and is big enough to stand on without teetering. Now, while you're listening to the news on the radio in the morning, step up and down at a regular beat, counting for two seconds up and two down, for two hundred times. Needless to say, you shouldn't start at two hundred. Start at thirty and work up to the big number. The step-box will start your arteries tingling long before you hit the shower.

The basis of any activity program is the realization that man was put on earth to walk. If he had been designed to run or jog, then most likely he would have been born with hooves. But walking, nature's way of maintaining your level of activity, is the closet activity of the decade. Some people have to take clandestine walks after dark. Their North American neighbors don't see that they are deliberately not on wheels, and are not reduced to walking, but are walking to reduce.

Not that strolling is forgotten all over the world. Europeans

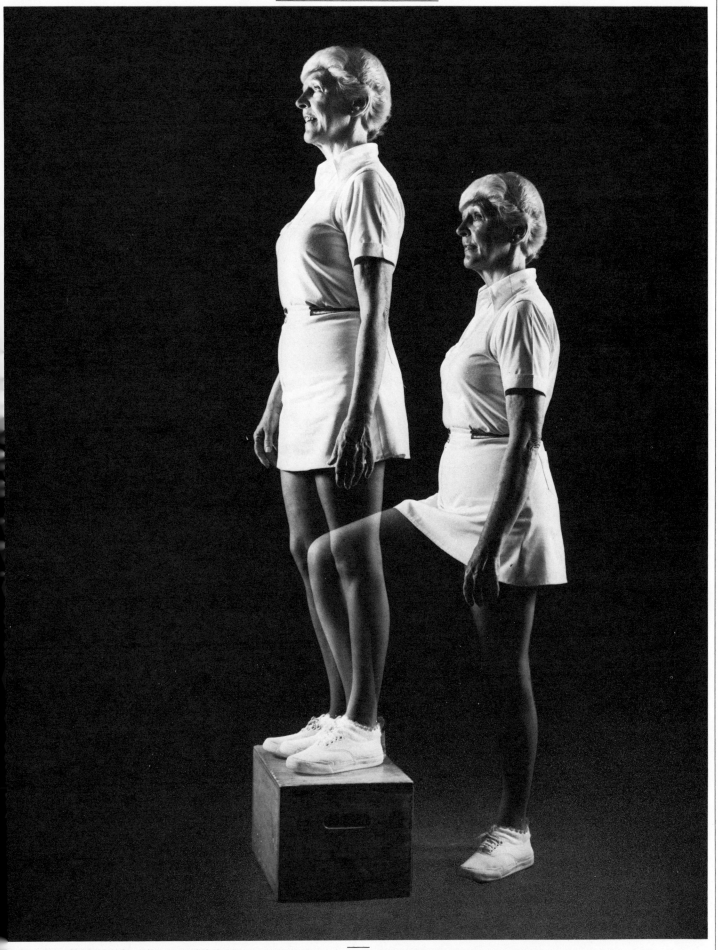

still rate walking as a highly desirable, effective, social activity. However, you don't just get out and walk! No, it's necessary to do a little preparation.

In the first place, there are several different ways of walking. Begin walking slowly, shaking your hands, letting your shoulders move as freely as possible. This is a warming-up process. Walking is not simply a matter of sauntering along and counting the sparrows on the telephone wire. This can be enjoyable but should be part of the cooling-down process rather than the actual hard-core pedestrianism. Once you're warmed up, see if you can spin the world. At the end of your stride, just as you're coming to the part where you push yourself off the ground, give a little extra shove as though you were trying to spin the world backwards under your feet. When you have developed high walking skills, then you can actually feel the world move a little bit as you push off!

While your feet are well designed for walking, the pavements aren't. This means you have to give some thought to shoes. A thick-soled pair of shoes is best if you are walking in the country, on grass or on rough ground. They prevent you from picking up stone bruises. In the city a pair of well-padded sneakers is best. Buy sneakers, not running shoes, so that you won't be peer-pressured into marathoning. The heel-counter of the shoe should fit your heel closely to prevent any up and down scraping. There's no special advantage to negative heels. However, make sure the sole is shock-absorbent.

Of course, you can always progress from walking to something a little faster, jogging. However, this isn't recommended. Jogging or running frequently causes a good deal of high-impact jarring on your heels and can bring out problems in the knee, ankle or back. Actually, you can get all the energy output you need from simply walking along smartly.

And don't forget the pleasurable joys of hiking. A good Sunday hike, preferably through a green environment, can ease the frustrations of the week and is better than any medication, either prescribed or bottled. Make sure you swing your arms well forward to ensure lots of help with your deep breathing.

If you carry a walking stick, all the better. You can carry it at the trail, that is at right angles to your arm, or in the normal manner reaching out in front and spearing the ground. All sorts of flourishes which use up a few more calories can be added to the way you use your stick. Besides, it can also protect you against people in a hurry who forget you are entitled to a portion of the sidewalk.

Or you can try speed walking. Push yourself along as rapidly as possible, letting your hips slide out sideways, with your elbows bent to 90 degrees. Go as fast as you can, but remember to stay within the talk limit. If you are so short of breath that you can't talk, then you're pushing yourself too much, so slow down.

There was some discussion earlier about swimming. It's a first class activity and puts most of the body through a good range of movement, and for flexibility exercises, it is without peer. Endurance swimming, that is where you increase the time in the water on a regular basis, can do a great deal to build cardiovascular fitness. Do not get out of the water immediately after your long-range swim. Stand in the shallow end and do a cool-down routine of slowly moving your arms and legs through a full range of motion. However, let's face it, swimming can be dull. Unless there is some type of group activity in the pool, most people find they just can't do it as frequently as is necessary.

While you're in the water don't forget there are other exercises that can be done. Bobbing, where you stand chest-high in the pool and then bend your knees so that you bob up and down on the surface, can be a great way to develop your quadriceps. Try side stepping, when you are chest-high in the water. Stretch out one leg to the side as far as possible, and take big steps sideways. It builds muscles around the hip, which are necessary for balance. A good way to jog is in the pool using a flotation jacket. While standing upright in deep water, begin to jog. Although you exercise the jogging muscles, you avoid the damaging impact on the heel you sustain when jogging on land.

You may have to give some special attention to your ears. Plugs may be necessary as pool water can cause fungus infection. In addition, particularly when you're in a public pool, make sure that your eyes are well covered by swimmer's goggles to keep out the chlorine.

Skating, either on the ice or with rollers, is another road to increased well-being. Maintaining your level of fitness is a major problem during the cold, wet months. Skating and curling are two good means of calorie burning and muscle building. While you're at it, cross-country skiing combines all the advantages of jogging with none of the disadvantages of injuring your back or knees.

Actually there are few sports that are not good for you. Some present difficulties, particularly if you need to perform rapid, balanced movements as in basketball. Generally speaking, any sport that involves hitting things heavily such as racquet ball should be avoided because of possible damage to the shoulder. This even includes table tennis, which can sometimes lead to self-inflicted injuries. However, if you are used to playing such games, by all means continue.

Golf is a great way to get some mobility in your back and at the same time maintain your level of physical fitness while doing a lot of walking. The problem with golfing is usually the associated nineteenth hole activity which may tear down all the good work you've built up in the previous three hours.

And don't forget dancing! There's some rhythm, you're doing it with somebody else so you're not likely to get bored, and it requires a lot of energy. In addition, it's good for developing balance, and as long as you don't try to be the belle of the ball while doing an overenthusiastic Hustle, then you will be O.K. Of course, if you're really energetic, square dancing or Scottish dancing (or that of any other nationality) can stir up old or tired blood vessels in a remarkable way.

The important thing is to give some thought to activities which can be done outside the exercise room.

Don't forget what can be one of the most important activities — sexercise. Certainly sexual activity can use a lot of energy and keep you mobile. The pulse rate usually goes above 120 for a short time. The snag is that most people feel that when they're in their sunset years, the flag has been lowered down the pole. Don't you believe it! Like any other physical activity, the law of use it or lose it holds. Some people are worried that it may be too violent an activity and can be dangerous, but that's simply not the case. Sexual activity, like any other physical activity, is a normal and healthy pastime after fifty.

While doing most of these activities you should check your heart rate as described on pages 14 and 20.

• ● •

Energy fitness depends on how active you are and the number of calories you eat. To maintain a reasonable weight level it is necessary to spend all the calories taken in. You can keep a rough balance of your daily status by comparing deposits with expenditures.

A normal diet, with only small servings of dessert and taking it easy with the sugar in the coffee and one small drink without mixer can run up about 3500 calorie intake.

Basic living activities, just breathing and thinking, use about 1500. So you need to spend 2000 more. Well, some general activities use calories as can be seen in the following table.

Calories used per minute

Standing	1.6	Walking-slowly	2.8
Ironing Clothes	4.2	-normal pace	4.4
Gardening	5.8	-quickly	5.1
Bedmaking	5.3	Cycling	6.7
Stair climbing	7.6	Dancing	5.7

From these figures it is obvious that it's necessary to keep busy all day and in addition do some exercise, if you wish to live on the credit side of your caloric checking account.

———————— • ● • ————————

All of this talk about swimming pools and halls where you can get together with your group and do something about physical fitness highlights the necessity for doing something about making more facilities available. While thousands of ice hockey rinks and other sport activity centers are built for the younger members of our society, there's little public property that has been made available with the over-fifty citizen in mind. Yes, there are tea rooms or bingo parlors or lawn bowling greens; however, special facilities which are dedicated to older citizens rather than young athletes are strangely lacking.

But they aren't really lacking. They're out there. All you have to do is to turn them up. Many communities have swimming pools where, after suitable negotiations, arrangements can be made for a time when beginners get in, get wet and get fit. Many hospitals have gymnasiums which are silent from 5 P.M. to 9 A.M. Community centers, which are a beehive of buzzing activity by elite athletes at certain times of the day, can be rescheduled to make sure that someone who's just in the early stages of the fitness game can do his thing without being knocked over in the rush.

All you have to do is make your wishes known, in no uncertain language, and develop these areas for your specific needs.

———————— • ● • ————————

Now, you have a plan. The exercises are safe and sane. There's room for change and for finding new pleasures in new activities. There's no need to get caught up in some fanatical desire to run across Boston or spend the best part of the day chasing some retreating goal set down by a frustrated decathalon director.

You're ready to join the fitness after fifty brigade. Enjoy it!

PROGRESS CHART

Day	WEEK ONE				WEEK TWO				WEEK THREE				WEEK FOUR			
	Flexibility	Energy	Special	Resting Heart Rate	Flexibility	Energy	Special	Resting Heart Rate	Flexibility	Energy	Special	Resting Heart Rate	Flexibility	Energy	Special	Resting Heart Rate
SUNDAY	1, 2, 3, 4, 5, 6, 8, 9, 10, 11	7 plus a walk														
MONDAY	1, 2, 3, 4, 5, 6, 8, 9, 10, 11															
TUESDAY	1, 2, 3, 4, 5, 6, 8, 9, 10, 11	7 plus a walk														
WEDNESDAY	1, 2, 3, 4, 5, 6, 8, 9, 10, 11															
THURSDAY	1, 2, 3, 4, 5, 6, 8, 9, 10, 11	7 plus a walk														
FRIDAY	1, 2, 3, 4, 5, 6, 8, 9, 10, 11															
SATURDAY	1, 2, 3, 4, 5, 6, 8, 9, 10, 11															

*See page 19 for instructions

PROGRESS CHART*

	WEEK FIVE				WEEK SIX				WEEK SEVEN				WEEK EIGHT			
	Flexibility	Energy	Special	Resting Heart Rate	Flexibility	Energy	Special	Resting Heart Rate	Flexibility	Energy	Special	Resting Heart Rate	Flexibility	Energy	Special	Resting Heart Rate
SUNDAY																
MONDAY																
TUESDAY																
WEDNESDAY																
THURSDAY																
FRIDAY																
SATURDAY																

PROGRESS CHART

	WEEK NINE			WEEK TEN			WEEK ELEVEN			WEEK TWELVE		
	Flexibility	Energy	Special	Resting Heart Rate	Flexibility	Energy	Special	Resting Heart Rate	Flexibility	Energy	Special	Resting Heart Rate	
SUNDAY													
MONDAY													
TUESDAY													
WEDNESDAY													
THURSDAY													
FRIDAY													
SATURDAY													

*See page 19 for instructions

PROGRESS CHART*

	WEEK THIRTEEN			WEEK FOURTEEN			WEEK FIFTEEN			WEEK SIXTEEN		
	Flexibility	Energy	Special	Resting Heart Rate	Flexibility	Energy	Special	Resting Heart Rate	Flexibility	Energy	Special	Resting Heart Rate
SUNDAY												
MONDAY												
TUESDAY												
WEDNESDAY												
THURSDAY												
FRIDAY												
SATURDAY												

About the Authors

Charles Godfrey, B.A., M.A., M.D., F.R.C.P.(C)
Dr. Godfrey is a well-known specialist in the care of senior citizens.
He is the Director of Rehabilitation Medicine at Wellesley Hospital in
Toronto and a Professor of Rehabilitation Medicine at the University
of Toronto. The author of three books and many articles in newspapers,
magazines and medical journals, he is a frequent guest on national
television programs in the health and fitness fields.

Michael Feldman, B.A., B.Ed.
Michael Feldman, a fitness consultant who specializes in working
with older people, is the Director of Wellness for the Racquet Sports
Group of Canada. A popular guest on television and radio, he is also a
frequent guest speaker at conferences. He has run many successful clinics
using the exercises in *The Ageless Exercise Plan*.